Antimicrobial Resistance

Jose L. Garcia, MD

Wade H. Melvin. AAFP Diplomat

Naomi F Melvin, PhD

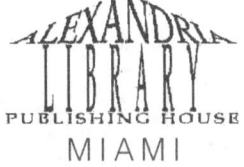

ALEXANDRIA LIBRARY
PUBLISHING HOUSE
MIAMI

Antimicrobials are, in many cases, the entire
visible part of a deeper problem.

The author

TABLE OF CONTENT

PREFACE

Communicable diseases are now the leading cause of death among children and young adults, mainly in third world countries. They cause more than thirteen million deaths and more than half of these occur in developing countries.

According to WHOM, these represent 45% of all deaths in poor countries, and 60% of deaths in children 0 -4 years worldwide. Acute respiratory infections, AIDS, EDA, TB, Malaria and measles are the main. Social deprivation, poverty concerns determine the world today, affecting one of the main human rights. The right to health

today are more resistant germs and complicated mechanisms and human faces a fight by decreasing the resistance offered by the microorganisms and their most effective weapon is not in sophisticated laboratories or complex chemical reactions, is in its rationality to efficiently use the weapons it owns in this fight. Antimicrobial

Pediatrics is one of the medical specialties where the use of antimicrobials is one of the most common prescriptions in clinical practice. It is known that children are more vulnerable to infection and its consequences for the weakened capacity for self-defense in this age group, which causes a morbidity and mortality in children less than one year.

WHO reports indicate that at least half of use antimicrobials, whether in the community and in hospitals, it is unnecessary and inappropriate. We have faith that this modest work serves to give out, plus all the scientific value that it holds itself, proper and rational use of these drugs and thus help reduce bacterial resistance; and most worrying is that it is growing every day. You need to save one of the great achievements of medicine: The discovery and subsequent development of antimicrobial drugs. This could mean saving the existence, since this resistance is the "Silent epidemic of the century".

We are sure that our students and faculty of different levels will appreciate how important therapeutic and rational control in infectious diseases.

Chapter   1

OVERVIEW OF THE THERAPEUTIC ANTIMICROBIAL

The constant struggle of man to achieve each day better health has faced, from time immemorial, a large number of microorganisms, many of which are life threatening.

The relentless war against these germs has come to this day, despite having in our therapeutic arsenal with numerous drugs capable of destroying, or at least reduce pathogenic cell populations to a size that can be controlled by the host immune mechanisms discovery, development and clinical application antimicrobials is considered one of the greatest advances in the field of therapeutic because it allowed a radical change in the morbidity and mortality of infectious diseases. However, the synthesis of this large amount of antimicrobials, especially in recent decades, has introduced a new and worrisome problem. The significant increases in antimicrobial resistance germs have become resistant to many of the agents intended to combat such result of chromosomal, or through the exchange of genetic material changes. But man does not cease in its efforts to emerge victorious in this new battle front.

The successful treatment of infectious diseases is the result of a complex process that depends on the interaction of many interrelated factors:

1. **By the causative organism:**
   a) Type microorganism
   b) Antimicrobial susceptibility
   c) Microbial resistance
   d) Kinetics of growth

2. **For the antimicrobial:**
   a) Family or pharmacological group
   b) Antimicrobial spectrum
   c) Pharmacokinetics
   d) Dosage
   e) Duration of treatment
   f) Pharmacodynamics

g) Efficacy / safety / cost

h) Associations

3. For the host:

a) Location of infection

b) Conditions of the infecting focus

c) Special therapeutic problems:

- Physiological (Age, pregnancy, lactation)

- Pathological (trauma or invasive procedures that alter the body's natural defense systems, immunosuppression, failure kidney, liver failure, severity of infection, etc.)

One of the major strategies of the modern pharmaceutical industry is the creation of drugs that act by blocking the increasing resistance of microorganisms to antimicrobial, either by beta-lactamase inhibitors (BLI), by creating new molecules or modifying existing ones. In all cases the aim is to prevent the activity of these enzymes responsible for resistance.

The investigations focus today its purposes in the pursuit of the ideal antibiotic. Which would have to respond favorably to a group of features among which are:

1. Pharmacodynamics:

- Possess bactericidal activity against the widest possible pathogens systems
- Be stable to beta-lactamases
- Not have effects side significant on organ and to present these effects are minimized.

2. Pharmaceutical:

- Be available in liquid forms
- Possess a pleasant taste
- That can be administered with food

3. Pharmacokinetic:

- Possess a prolonged half-life scale,
- Good penetration in fluids body maintain concentrations required to inhibit bacterial replication
- That is not metabolized, and that when this happens can participate in drug interactions
- Make it eliminated renal through glomerular filtration.

- Possess low toxicity.

4. **Economic.**
   - Patient Affordability

The search is not over the objectives are plotted, the resources are available, human intelligence is working at full capacity. With all this you can glimpse the future.

Once again the battle for life is raised and there is no doubt that man will gracefully, but there are still obstacles to overcome ... The human knowledge should be passed from generation to generation, progress and achievements that are achieved should be made available to all and not in the hands of a few, intelligence must be devoted to control and not to create new and powerful germs in sophisticated laboratories. Only then we will win this war, death, life. Therefore vital importance the constant updating of our doctors, who must be familiar with all these aspects Chemotherapy.

ANTIMICROBIAL CHEMOHERAPY: ORIGINS

One concept that revolutionized scientific thinking and ushered in the current development of modern antimicrobial chemotherapy was by Paul Ehrlich formulation of the principles of selective toxicity in the first decade of the twentieth century. He showed that there were substances that can be harmful to a parasite and harmless to the host and conducted experiments with arsenic which also considered the first major triumph of chemotherapy, allowed the initial recognition of the specific relationships that occur between parasites and drugs.

On this fundamental principle of selective toxicity based antimicrobial therapy to destroy a pathogenic cell population (bacteria, fungi, protozoa, etc.) or reduce it to such a size that can be controlled by the host immune mechanisms.

DEFINITIONS

Antimicrobials are able with their action to destroy these populations and thus cause lysis and death of the germ are called **bactericides;** those that inhibit bacterial growth and thus reduce the pathogenic cell populations are considered **bacteriostatic** poses.

Starting is currently the era of antimicrobial chemotherapy in 1935, with the emergence of sulfonamides and antibiotic therapy with the use of penicillin, discovered by Alexander Fleming since 1929.

Initially these drugs were isolated from filtered media in which fungi producers had grown. Over the years and due to the development of other sciences, it has been passed to the biosynthetic modification of molecules. That is why earlier to drugs used to fight infections were known variously as **antibiotics** when they were made from natural and microorganisms **chemotherapeutic** when they were produced by chemical synthesis. However, and to avoid misconceptions were called **antimicrobial** drug naturally occurring, semisynthetic or synthetic used to suppress the growth of microorganisms and eventually cause death.

ANTIMICROBIALS CLASSIFICATION

Antimicrobial drugs are constituted by very different kinds of compounds and are often classified into groups or families for these features. On the other hand, it is also common to find classifications that divide them according to their antibacterial spectrum, as the effect of their action, according to their mechanism of action on bacteria, according to their chemical structure, etc. Therefore it is difficult to determine which is the ideal, but the fact is that each provides basic information relevant to your knowledge and use families.

Classification of antimicrobials by groups or

I. Aminocyclitols	Espectinomicina
II. Aminoglycosides	Streptomycin, neomycin, kanamycin, gentamicin, tobramycin, amikacin, Dibekacin, Netilmicin.

III. Betalactams
  a) Penicillin

• Benzylpenicillins Phenoxymethylpenicillin	Penicillin G (Crystal, procaine, benzathine)
• Aminopenicillins	Ampicillin, Amoxicillin
• Isoxazoxilpenicilinas	oxacillin, cloxacillin, methicillin, nafcillin
• Carboxypenicillins	Carbenicillin, Ticarcillin, Carfenicilina
• Ureidopenicillins	Azlocillin, Mezlocillin, Piperacillin, Alpacilina

  b) Cephalosporins

• 1st generation	Cephalexin, Cefazolin, cephalothin, Cefadroxil
• 2nd generation	Cefonocid, cefamandole, cefoxitin, Cefuroxime
• 3rd generation	Cefotetan, cefotaxime, ceftazidime, ceftriaxone
• 4th generation	Cefepime, Cefpirome

c) Carbapenems	imipenem, meropenem
d) monobactams	Aztreonam, carumonam, Tigemonan
e) inhibitors beta-lactamase(IBL)	clavulanic acid, sulbactam, tazobactam
IV. Diaminopyridines	Trimethoprim, Metioprima, pyrimethamine
V. streptogramins,	Pristinamycin virginiamycin, Quinopristina / Dalfopristin
VI. Phenicols	Chloramphenicol, Thiamphenicol
VII. Fosfomycins	Fosfocina, phosmidomicine
VIII. Fusidanos	fusidic acid
IX. Glycopeptides	vancomycin, Teicloplanina, Ramoplanin
X. Licosaminas	Lincomycin, Clindamycin
XI. Imidazoles	miconazole, ketoconazole, fluconazole
XII. Macrolides	Erythromycin Oleandomycin, Josamycin, Roxithromycin, azithromycin, clarithromycin
XIII. Nitroimidazoles	metronidazole, tinidazole, Ornidazol, Secnidazole
XIV. Nitrofuran	nitrofurantoin, nitrofurazone, furazolidone
XV. Antiviral nucleotide	Acyclovir, Vidarabine, cytarabine, Zidovudine
XVI. Polyenes	Nystatin, Amphotericin B
XVII. Polypeptides	polymyxin B, colistin, bacitracin

XVIII.quinolones

• 1st generation	nalidixic acid, oxolinic acid, Cinoxacin, pipemidicAcid
• 2nd generation	ciprofloxacin, norfloxacin, ofloxacin, enoxacin
• 3rd generation	temafloxacin, Difloxacin, Lomefloxacin

XIX. Rifamycins	rifampin, rifampin, Rifaxcimen
XX. Sulfone	Dapsone
XXI. Sulfonamides	sulfacetamide, mafenide, sulfasalazine, phthalyl Sulfathiazole, sulfadiazine, sulfisoxazole, Sulfimetoxazol, Sulfadoxine
XXII. Tetracyclines	chlortetracycline, tetracycline, doxycycline, minocycline

Classification of antimicrobials by action:

1. Bactericides:
   - Beta-lactam
   - Aminoglycosides
   - Glycopeptides
   - Rifamycines
   - Quinolones
   - Cotrimoxazol
   - Fosfomicina
   - Nitrofurans
2. Bacteriostatic:
   - Phenicols
   - lincosamides
   - macrolides
   - tetracyclines
   - sulfa

Classification according to the antibacterial action spectrum:

1. <u>Mainly against Gram positive bacteria:</u>
   - Benzylpenicillins
   - 1st generation cephalosporins
   - Glycopeptides
   - Macrolides
   - Lincosamides
   - Rifamycines
   - Bacitracin
   - Fusidic acid
2. <u>Mainly against Gram negative:</u>
   - Aminoglycosides
   - Monobactams
   - Polymyxins
3. <u>Broad spectrum:</u>
   - Aminopenicillins
   - Carboxypenicillins
   - Ureidopenicillins
   - Cephalosporins 2nd, 3rd and 4th generation
   - Carbapenems
   - Phenicols
   - Quinolones
   - Cotrimoxazol
   - Tetracyclines
4. <u>Against Germs anaerobios:</u>
   - Penicilinas
   - Cefoxitina
   - Carbapenémicos
   - Metronidazol
   - Fenicoles
   - Macrólidos
   - Lincosamidas

ACTION ANTIMICROBIAL MECHANISMS

If we stick to the principles enunciated by Ehrlich, an ideal antimicrobial agent should show selective toxicity. Actually this term is relative ... they often do a drug in a given concentration is tolerable to the host but can harm the infectious agent is present.

This principle clearly understand when analyzing the mechanisms of action using antimicrobials to act on infectious agents. Antimicrobial drugs exploit existing differential characteristics between the cells of the causative agents of infection and the host.

The target sites or receptors which exert their antimicrobial action may be cellular structures or biochemical reactions essential for the infectious agent, not white exist in the mammalian cell, or if there are, the more vulnerable the microorganism.

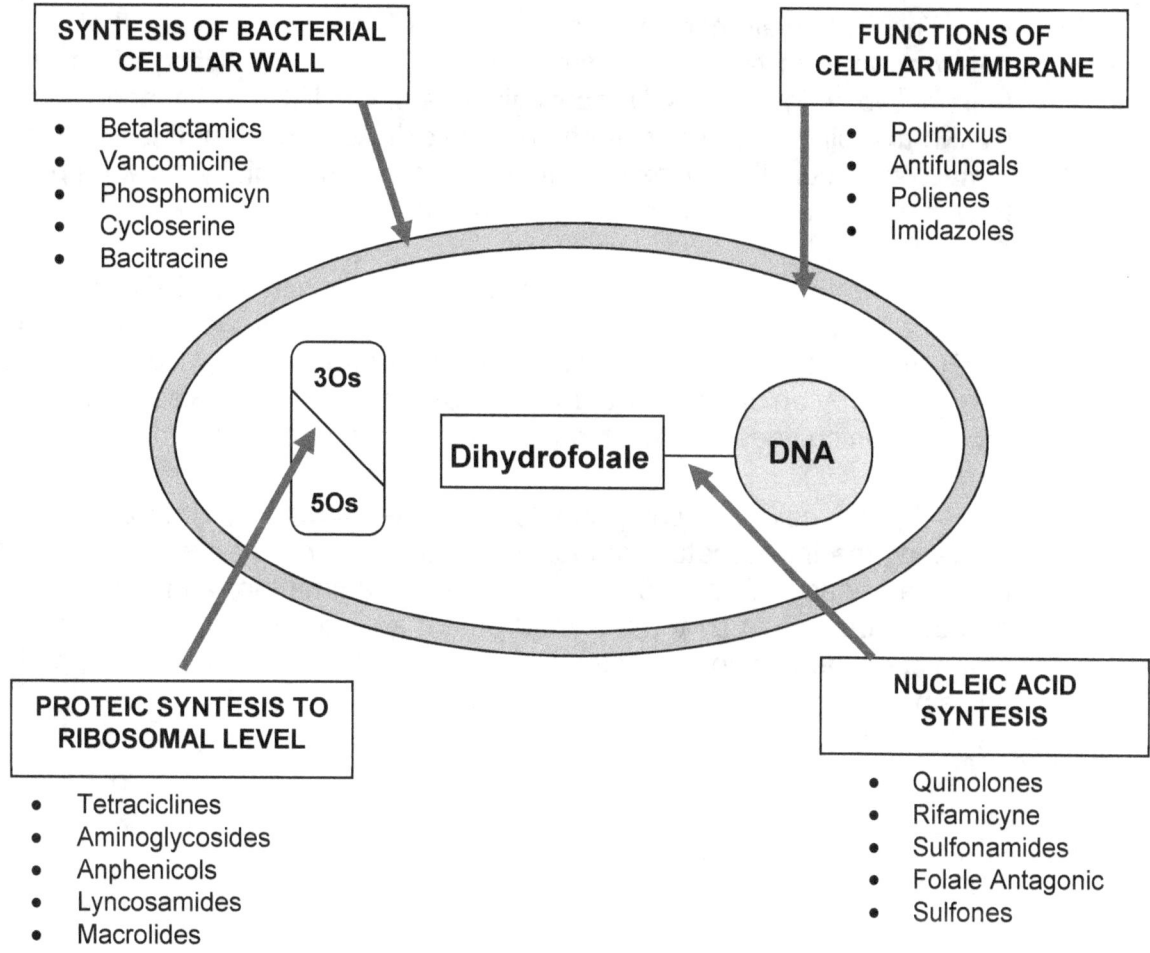

SYNTESIS OF BACTERIAL CELULAR WALL
- Betalactamics
- Vancomicine
- Phosphomicyn
- Cycloserine
- Bacitracine

FUNCTIONS OF CELULAR MEMBRANE
- Polimixius
- Antifungals
- Polienes
- Imidazoles

PROTEIC SYNTESIS TO RIBOSOMAL LEVEL
- Tetraciclines
- Aminoglycosides
- Anphenicols
- Lyncosamides
- Macrolides

NUCLEIC ACID SYNTESIS
- Quinolones
- Rifamicyne
- Sulfonamides
- Folale Antagonic
- Sulfones

30s

50s

Dihydrofolale

DNA

Fig. 1.1 Mechanism of action on the antimicrobials

1. Antimicrobials which inhibit cell wall synthesis Germ:

The bacteria, both Gram positive and Gram negative bacteria have an anatomical configuration quite similar. Their main bodies are covered by the much needed for them because the cell wall internal osmotic concentration of the bacterial cell is several times greater than that in the tissue fluid of mammals; so if this structure did not exist, the organisms quickly explode and die.

While living bacteria, the cell wall is constantly being synthesized in some areas and in others, simultaneously being lysed by autolytic enzymes (Acetilmuramiclasas) allowing you to renew its structure and cell division experience. If this synthesis is stopped, the balance would be broken and may be kept lysis resulting in the production of deficient forms wall (protoplast) to undergo lysis in an unprotected osmotically medium.

The cell wall consists of a layer of peptide glycan that it is a heteropolymer of two chains dimensional structure consisting of alternating units of two amino sugars: N- acetylglucosamine (NAG) and N-acetylmuramic (NAM) that bind small peptide chains by acid. As a result of this crosslinking, a macromolecule that gives stability and mechanical rigidity allowing bacteria to withstand the osmotic pressure remaining.

One of the structural differences between positive and Gram negative bacteria it is precisely the configuration of their cell wall. Peptide glycan layer of Gram-negative bacteria is thinner than in Gram positive bacteria, being surrounded by an outer membrane of phospholipids, lipopolysaccharides and proteins; which does not occur in Gram positive where the lipid layer is thicker.

These cell wall components of bacteria play an important role in triggering the inflammatory response because they are able to trigger it and produce release of chemical mediators of inflammation, although the germ has been destroyed by the action of potent antimicrobial that we have today stages peptide glycan biosynthesis enzymes and involves 30 is divided into three basic

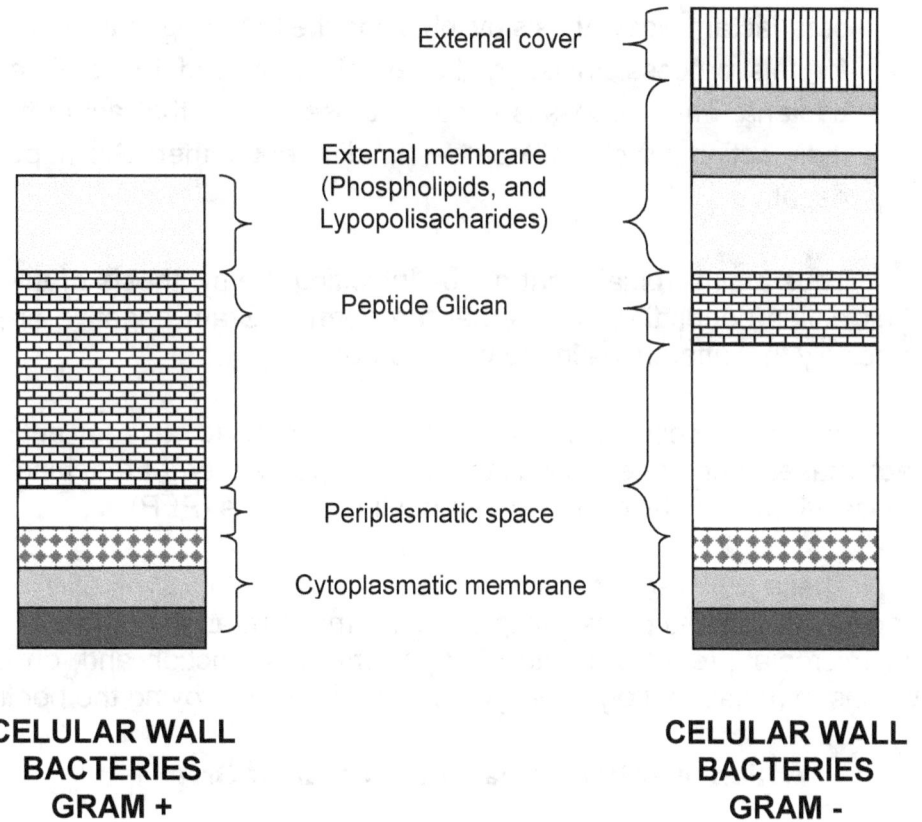

External cover

External membrane
(Phospholipids, and
Lypopolisacharides)

Peptide Glican

Periplasmatic space

Cytoplasmatic membrane

**CELULAR WALL
BACTERIES
GRAM +**

**CELULAR WALL
BACTERIES
GRAM -**

- **First stage:**
  It occurs in the cytoplasm and its PARK to nucleotide product. It pentapeptide primary units are joined. This stage is inhibited by D-cycloserine which interrupts the last reaction thereof: racemization of L-alanine and for the condensation catalyst D-ala-D-ala synthetase consequently the bacterium lacks the basic formative elements for develop wall.

- **Second stage**
  Involves PARK nucleotide binding with uridine diphosphate-acetyl glucosamine to form linear cords cell wall material called glycans peptides which must cross the cell membrane and arranged in the increasing wall. At this stage the complete unit is separated cytoplasmic membrane phospholipids. This reaction is inhibited by vancomycin stage.

- **Third stage**
  Includes transpeptidation reaction that occurs outside the cytoplasmic membrane and produces the full crossover between the two chains to form a structure of increased rigidity, similar to a fishing net. At this level of acting

beta-lactam biosynthesis by inhibiting the transpeptidase enzyme responsible for this process, initiating the events that lead to death and lysis of the bacteria. This process is used by those agents that act at this level to exert their action which, of course, is different either Gram positive or Gram negative.

Thus antimicrobials that act by inhibiting the synthesis of this wall, carry out their action depending on whether the germ is Gram negative or positive, taking precisely the differences in the wall thereof.

In Gram positive bacteria, that manage to evade antimicrobial beta-lactamases, penetrate the wall through the pores thereof reaching the periplasmic space where they bind to penicillin-binding proteins (PFP).

These PFP are responsible for catalyzing the synthesis of the precursor peptide glycan and crosslinking to the normal formation of the wall, so to join them antimicrobial prevents him to PFP perform this function and, on the other hand, begins to release autolytic enzymes capable of destroying the peptide glycan.

Action of antimicrobials on the wall of Gram +

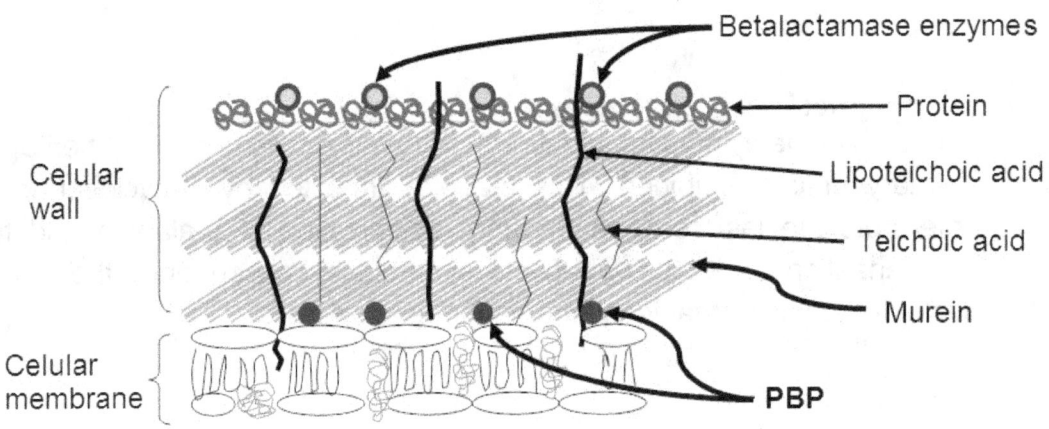

PBP   Penicillin-binding protein

By these two methods, variants is then synthesized abnormal wall that does not have the ability to withstand the osmotic pressure which results in that the bacteria explode and die.

However, in the Gram negative bacteria, this function cannot be fulfilled so easily, due to the characteristics of the cell wall in them.

In Gram negative, the outer layer of lipopolysaccharides and phospholipids is a very efficient barrier to the antimicrobial action. When these drugs pass through the pores of this structure are attacked by beta-lactamases, strategically located in the periplasmic space and cannot get to join the PFP in order to fulfill its action of inhibiting the synthesis of the peptide glycan and therefore bacterial achieved survive.

Antimicrobial Action on the wall of Gram -

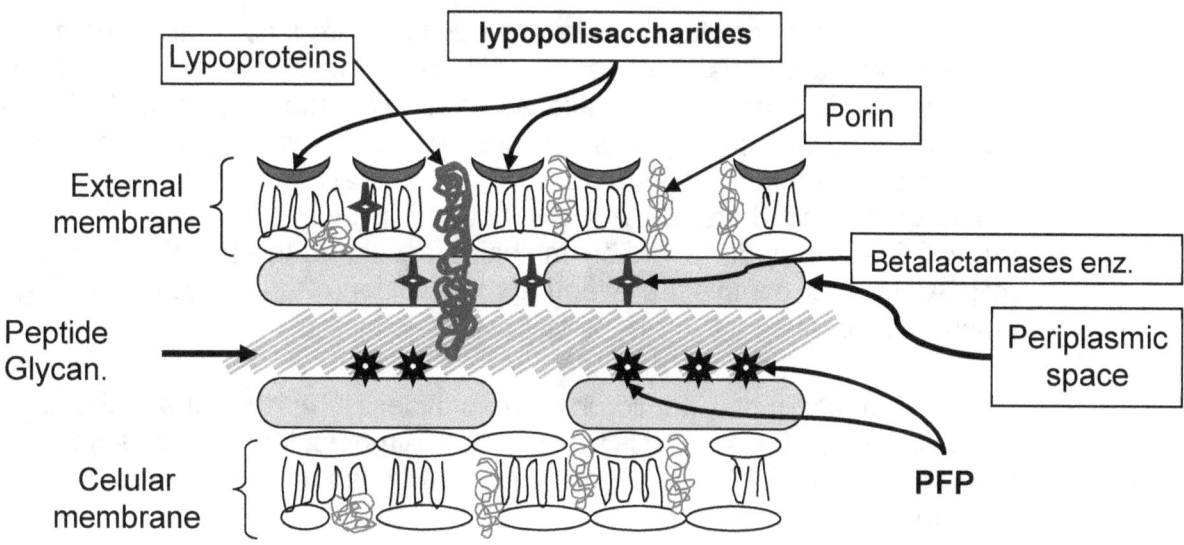

2. Antimicrobials that inhibit protein synthesis at the ribosomal level:

Ribosomes are rich in RNA granules have been in the endoplasmic reticulum and are involved in protein synthesis. Bacteria have ribosomes 70s, whereas mammalian cells have ribosomes 80s.

The synthesis of proteins in a living cell is a complex process dependent DNA core to establish the amino acid sequence and thus be able to secrete proteins synthesized. The direction of discharge from the DNA includes transcription or DNA code decoding in a disposable mRNA molecule then moves to the cytoplasm where his formation results in the production of proteins by ribosomes. Bacteria possess polysomes, which are able to read ribosome mRNA message is strung along the strip mRNA.

In this simplified form, one can see the importance of these structures for maintaining cell life. In this case, the bacterial cell.

The ribosomes of bacteria are sufficiently different as to the sub-units that comprise their chemical composition and their functional specificities, which helps explain why antimicrobials that inhibit Bacteria do not have the greatest effect on animal cells.

Antimicrobial acting at this level binds to different sub-units that make up the ribosome and thus can interfere with this vital cellular process, ensuring their bactericidal or bacteriostatic as case. For example, bind to the 30S ribosomal subunit: aminoglycosides interrupting at least the first step of protein synthesis (reaction initiation), resulting in formation of abnormal complex: monosomes and therefore not a functional protein also join this sub-unit tetracycline's; they do reversibly inhibiting access to the site tRNA ribosomal mRNA acceptor complex, preventing the addition of amino acids forming the polypeptide chain.

In the case of antimicrobial macrolides type the 50s subunit bind reversibly, when the subunit is free from tRNA molecules, thereby suppressing the production of highly polymerized unaffected homopeptides the small peptide.

Chloramphenicol also acts on the subunit to bind reversibly to this portion to inhibit bacterial protein synthesis by blocking the formation of peptide bonds by inhibiting dipeptidyl - transferase and similarly prevent the binding of aminoacyl - tRNA to the ribosome. Lincomycins perform the same action on the 50S sub unit emphasize, is necessary to finally, all of these drugs to exert their action necessarily have to pass through the membrane in several ways: transported through complex energy dependent processes, oxidative phosphorylation and cellular respiration; by passive diffusion; through the hydrophilic membrane pores; by facilitated diffusion, etc.

3. Antimicrobials which inhibit the permeability of the cell membrane

The cytoplasm of all living cells is surrounded by the cytoplasmic membrane, which serves as a barrier perm selective performs functions of active transport, and thus controls the internal composition of the cell.

This membrane has a basic structure trilaminar chemically composed of phospholipids, protein and a small amount of carbohydrates which gives a thickness of 75-180 nm. If the functional integrity of the cytoplasmic membrane is interrupted escape protein and purine and pyrimidine nucleotides, which results in cell damage and death.

These features are leveraging drugs like amphotericin B, colistin or polymyxin Nystatin to exert its selective antimicrobial action, to behave as cationic detergent and attack conjugation sites it.

Antimicrobial action on the cytoplasmic membrane

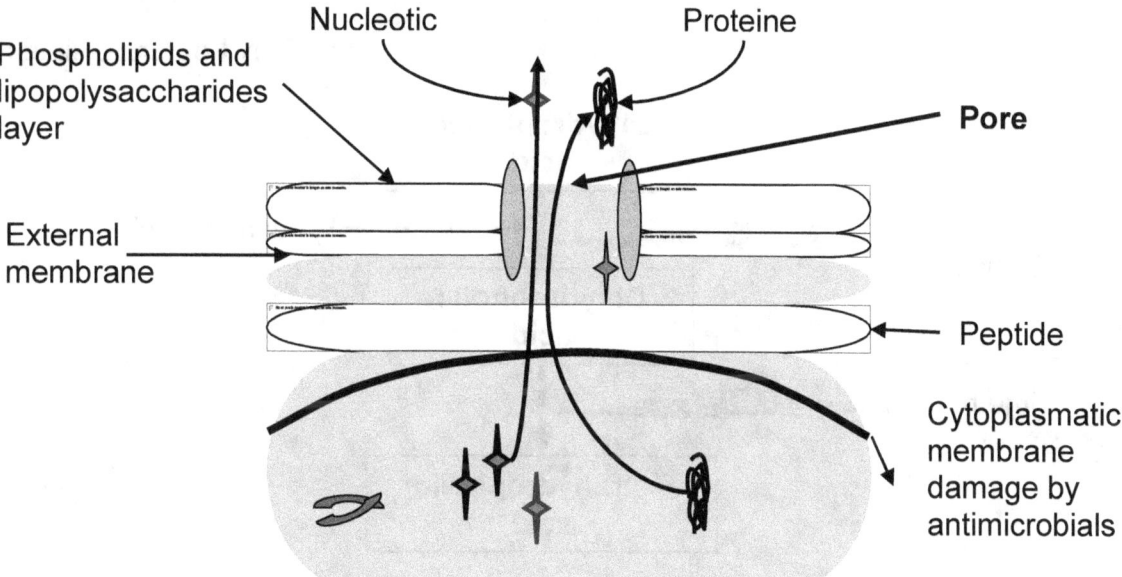

4. Antimicrobial affecting nucleic acid synthesis

For many microorganisms the para-amino benzoic acid (PABA) is an essential metabolite. It is used as a precursor of folic acid, which serves as an important step in the synthesis of nucleic acids.

The specific mode of action of PABA involves ATP, condensation of a protein energy dependent with PABA to produce dihydropteroic which is subsequently converted to folic acid. Antimicrobial sulfonamides use their structural analogy with PABA to penetrate the reaction competing for the active site of the enzyme. As a result, they form similar non-functional folate which prevents further development of the bacterial cell.

Action as antimetabolites about germs

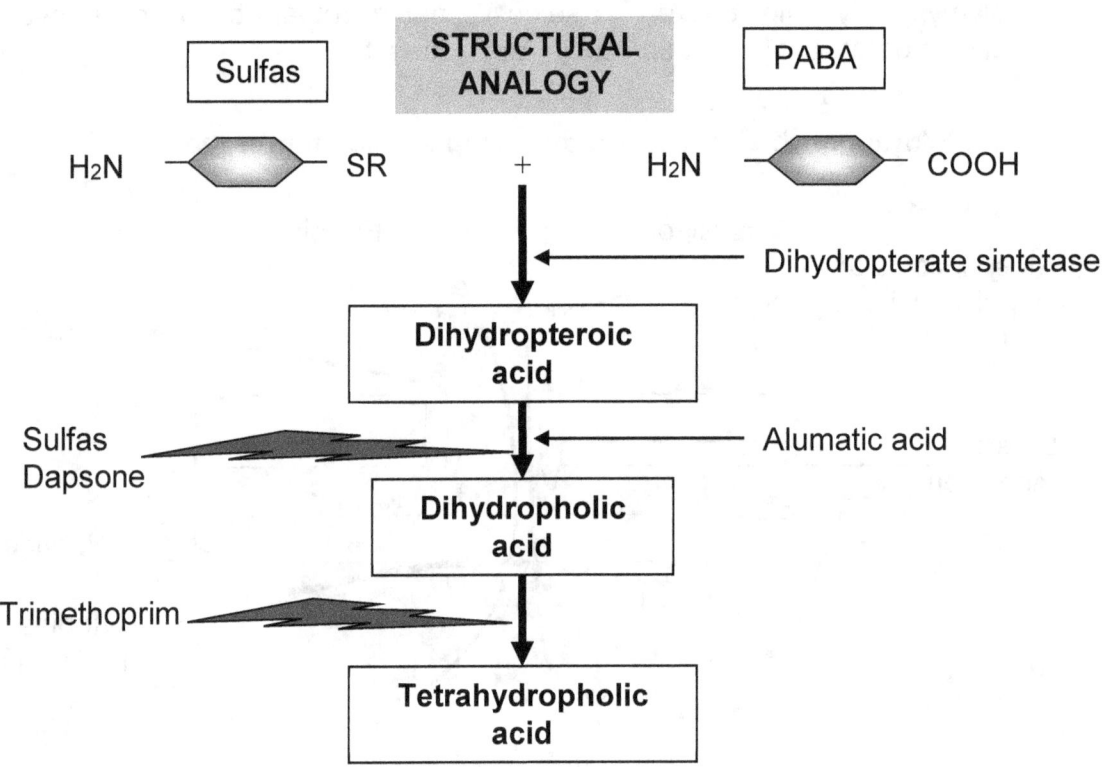

Ropin and pyrimethamine are inhibitors potentially dihydrofolate reductase and have been sulfonamides mixed with achieving a marked synergism in their antimicrobial activity. And then, separately, and trimethoprim sulfa have a bacteriostatic effect; but to join in a single product (cotrimoxazole) synergism with marked bactericidal effect is achieved.

Also in this category those drugs that have a mechanism of action directly linked to the inhibition of RNA polymerase-dependent DNA, vital enzyme to include the cell to produce mRNA using standard DNA as template. Rifampicin, quinolones and nitrofurantoin have an action that is included in the inhibition of DNA-gyrase.

REFERENCES

1. Jacqz-Aigrain, Choonara I. Editors. Paediatric Clinical Pharmacology.
    a. Ed. Taylor & Francis.2006.
2. GM Morejon current infectious Panorama. RESUMED 9 (3): 139-144,
    a. 1996.
3. Murray PR Medical microbiology. The 4th ed. Ed. Mosby. Vol. 4: 195-395,
    a. 2002.
4. Goodman and Bilman. Pharmacological Basis of Therapeutics. Vol II
    a. ed 9 (2):1996.
5. Monthly. Over antibiotic us. Prescribing references. Ed. Sales-Sataff. 188-
    a. 208, 2005.
6. Rudolph H. Antibacterial therapy.20th ed. Ed. Appleton and Lange. 444,
    a. 1996.
7. Llop H. Valdes-Dapena V. Ma. M. Ed Micobiology and medical parasitology. Ecimed. Volume I. 81-99, 2001.
8. Lieberman J Infect Dis J. M. Pediatric 22.11433, 2003.
9. Giving S A. Trains Biochem Sci. 29,159,2004.
10. S Sivagnanam, Deleu D. Critical care 7 119 2003.
11. Torres MJ, White M, Fernández J, et al. Allergy. 58,961,2003.
12. H. Nikaido Microbiol Mol Biol Rev. 67, 593, 2003.
13. Sanchez Garcia, JL, Varona, F. Antimicrobial, general considerations. ESCIMED edition, 2009

Chapter 2

Interrelations guest. - Bacterial infectious Parasite

The body has a complex system of recognition and antimicrobial defense That Allows it to survive DESPITE ITS With continuous interaction pathogens or microbes. Host defenses against pathogens require proper coordination of multiple effector pathways. These pathways are activated to the identification of microbial molecules produced, starting an inflammatory cascade That includes the recruitment of leukocytes to the site of the infection and activation of antimicrobial effector Mechanisms by way of second messengers; That an adaptive immune response Promotes elimination of infection and immune memory .

These defense systems include development of innate and adaptive immune responses Mechanisms mediated by T and B controls the host interactions - microbe. The end result of These interactions have a range from the symbiosis With the commensal microflora; asymptomatic or mild infections; to severe infectious diseases by highly virulent organisms, Depending on the particular host and the infecting organism par excellence phagocytes, Such as macrophages, neutrophils and dendritic cells are the only cell units qualifying for wrapping large particles, treats including microorganisms. Endocytosis and subsequent destruction of pathogens are key to the innate immune response, antigen presentation Promote and development of adaptive immunity. After antigenically marked, the organism is trapped in a vacuole derived from the periplasmic membrane.

The nascent phagosome must undergo a drastic conversion to acquire microbicides and degenerative properties that are associated with innate immunity. This known as phagosome maturation follows a strictly structured conversion of fission and fusion events involving the endocytic pathway defined compartments choreographic sequence. Effective phagocytosis requires two essential components: particle internalization and phagosome maturation recognition of the microorganism interaction with the phagocyte can be direct, through the phagocyte recognition of molecules associated with the pathogen receptor-mediated structure; or indirect, mediated opsoninas

Opsonins are host factors which are anchored to the surface of the pathogen, acquiring a spatial conformation which is recognized by receptors of the phagocyte, such as Fcɣ receptor (FcɣRs) and receptor C3 (C3R). The signal triggered by the particle varies depending on the nature of the receptor. Exposure to polyvalent ligands induces clustering of these receptors on the surface of the phagocyte membrane, initiating phosphorylation of its cytoplasmic immunoreceptor ITAMs by intracytoplasmic Kinases.

The immunoreceptor tyrosine phosphorylation activated recruits and activates the tyrosine kinase, which transforms on various substrates phosphorylated. In this process the remodeling of actin (Rac) is necessary for the issuance of pseudopodia, which in the particular case of FcɣR, polymerization is conducted by Rac1 / Rac2 and protein 42 control cell division.

Maturation phagosome begins immediately after possibly even before the phagosome be sealed, separated from the surface of the membrane, passes through a sequential phagosome fusion with early endosome, late endosome and lysosome. These steps ultimately lead to the formation of polifagosoma, which is the terminal state of the sequence of maturation and therefore the last microbicide organelle.

The polifagosoma is equipped with an array of complex and sophisticated mechanisms to eliminate microorganisms and degrade.

Microbicidal activity of the phagosome

Maturation sequence during the phagosome acquire an arsenal of microbicides determinates acidification.

- Phagosome: This creates a hostile environment that prevents bacterial growth and promotes action phagocyte numerous hydrolytic enzymes that act at acidic pH. Besides the transmembrane gradient hydrogen ions generated by the V - ATPase is used to inactivate and expel phagosome inside the microbial nutrients essential. The V - ATPase also facilitates the generation of superoxide radicalsintrafagosomicos.

- Reactive oxygen and nitrogen species: these reactive radicals synergize to exercise its highly toxic effect on microorganisms. The interaction of radicals with toxic components of microorganism inactivation result brings changes in proteins and lipids by oxidative damage. The microbial DNA suffers irreparable damage disrupts the bacterial metabolism and culminates in inhibiting replication.

- Antimicrobial peptides and protein. There are a group of proteins that can be divided into: the interfering bacterial growth (bacteriostatic) and that compromise the integrity of the microorganism (bactericidal). The bacteriostatic proteins limit the availability of essential nutrients within the phagosome. For this the secret phagocyte competing substances into the phagosome or inserted in the membrane active transporters. The first compete for nutrients and expel the latter inside the phagosome including:

For its part, the bactericidal are more direct mechanisms that displays the phagosome to destroy pathogenic organisms,

Defensins, cathelicidins, lysozyme, lipases and proteases. Defensins are divided into two groups α and ß are small polypeptides linked by disulfide bridges stored in primary granules. Its function is to induce membrane permeabilization of Gram positive and Gram negative bacteria by forming ion channels permeable multimeric. The activated cathelicidins permeabilize the cell wall and inner membrane of Gram positive bacteria and the inner and outer membrane of Gram-negative. Furthermore the phagosome is equipped with a number range endopeptidases, exopeptidases and hydrolases that degrade various microbial components.

Table 2.1 Peptides and proteins with antimicrobial activity.

Antimicrobial activity	Peptide or protein
Bacteriostatic nutrient	Lactoferrindeprivation.Faith kidnaps required for growth bacterial- NR AMP1 (associated protein 1 Macrophage natural resistance). Expulsion and uptake of divalent ions Fe, Zn, Mn.
Bactericides	
Membrane Permeabilization	Defensins cathelicidins
Hydrolysis • Carbohydrates • Lypids • Proteins Endopeptidases Exopeptidases	Lysozyme ß -glucuronidase Beta- hexosaminidase Phospholipase A$_2$ Cysteine proteases: cathepsins B, C, H, K, L, O, S and W. Aspartate Proteases: Cathepsins D and E Serine Proteases: Cathepsin G. carboxypeptidases: lysosomal carboxypeptidase A and B dipeptidase or cathepsin X, peptidyl - dipeptidase and prolilcarboxipeptidasa Aminopaptidasas.Cathepsin H; dipeptidylpeptidase I (captepsina C); tripeptidilpeptidasa dipeptidylpeptidase II and

Destructive bacterial phagocytosis resistance: mechanisms of bacterial evasion and escape the phagosome

Despite the presence of these antimicrobial factors, many pathogens can survive within host cells. Bacteria, fungi and viruses have developed multiple strategic mechanisms to counteract host defenses. Some bacterial species interfere with the ability of phagocytes to wrap them and form the phagosome; either by blocking, inhibiting or degradation antibody opsonization or complement system; fact that directly affects the phagocytic machinery macrophages, neutrophils and dendritic cells. Other bacteria have become resistant to one or more of the antimicrobial factors phagocyte and in some species have evolved metabolic pathways that counteract the accumulation of acid in the phagosome or acquired protein resistant to withstand the low pH. Bacteria which are actively degrading protect themselves antibacterial peptides and proteins produced by the phagocyte or through the production and activation of detoxifying enzymes such as catalase, which neutralizes toxic oxygen radicals and nitrogen or by recruitment of proteins which mediate synthesis these radicals. Certain bacterial species secrete molecules specialized in iron uptake, called sideroporos who kidnap and mark the cation to be used by the bacteria; finally many bacteria survive in the phagosome by developing a vigorous response to stress that lets you get rid or replace damaged proteins.

Escape of the phagosome.

The ability of intracellular survival is crucial for pathogenic bacteria, once they have invaded target cells. Either by the trigger mechanism or Zipper, it is internalized bacteria in a vacuole. Under normal conditions this vacuole acidified its internal environment progressively to the mature form degradative the phagolysosome. Many pathogens survive in its niche, avoiding the phagosome fusion -. Lysosome or by modifying the internal environment of the phagolysosome

Many of the mechanisms by which microorganisms survive and remain within the phagosome already been mentioned in the text. However, there are other, lesser known, through which bacteria acquire the ability to survive and replicate in the cytoplasm. Auminedo that the cytosol is a rich source of nutrients and is protected from immune destruction; one would expect that many bacteria could use the cytosol as a natural habitat for their growth and replication. However, only a select number of bacteria, have been adapted to grow in the cytosol. Examples are: *Shigella flexneri, Burkholderia pseudomallei, Listeria monocytogens, Rickettsia and Francisella tularensis*phases.

Cytoplasmic life cycle of the bacteria can be divided into three Escape from the vacuole, in the cytosol and replication blocking immune responses in cytosol vacuole.

- Escape Mechanisms of the Vacuola: The first step is crucial in the life cycle of pathogens cytosolic, is the exhaust from the vacuole. This occurs immediately after the invasion of the target cell. The speed with which the vacuolar lysis occurs suggests that the bacteria in a race for survival. The phagosome incipient acidified quickly and bacteria must escape before the phagosome fuses with the lysosome containing potent microbicidal compounds.

  All pathogens adopt the same strategy entry to the cytosol using based on the production and secretion of enzyme mechanisms, called protein bacterial escape.

  There are several mechanisms that are in place for the enzymatic lysis of the vacuole occurs. These enzymes are inserted into the thickness of the vacuole membrane, cholesterol binding to and forming pores that lead to membrane dysfunction. Thus phagosome maturation is delayed and prevents the lysosome fusion by alterations in the ion gradient across the membrane.

Rupture occurs vacuole and pathogens are free in the cytoplasm where they multiply and spread, infecting the neighboring cell; requiring this process to a set of enzymes. Escape mechanisms developed by pathogenic has the distinction of being own and unique to each gendercytosol.

- Bacterial replication in the Just a few bacteria, intracellular par excellence, they are able to survive and replicate in the cytoplasm. The entry of the bacteria in the bacterial phagocytic vacuole and subsequent escape seems to be a prerequisite for growth in the cytosol. The bacteria must first be packaged inside the phagosome to be ready for replication in the cytosol. The bacteria inside the phagosome starts the escape mechanism and releases enzymes that will create the conditions for growth in the cytosol. But the growth of bacteria in the cytosol depends on the cell type. This explains in part because cytosolic bacteria invade certain tissues of the body, perhaps related to different nutritional cytoplasmic requirements.

- Modulation or blocking the immune response Once the bacteria are included in the vacuole are outside the scope of the antibodies and complement. However, they are susceptible to degradation in the phagolysosome, which can be avoided if the bacteria escape the phagosome in the cytosol. And in the cytosol, the bacterium is not yet secure, because it contains several antimicrobial peptides and toxic oxygen radicals. In addition to this, the pathogens in the cytoplasm can not evade the immune response because they have on their surface molecules that are recognized by receptors that trigger specific intracytoplasmic inflammatory response. Another defense mechanism against pathogens is intracytoplasmic autophagy. This is a process in which the lysosomes causing cell death to maintain homeostasis. Therefore, it is required to survive a pathogen in the cytosol, it must interact and affect the properties of the cytosol own microbicides and autophagic route activity; currently has proposed the use of small cationic peptides with antimicrobial and immunomodulating they are virtually present in all life forms, as an important component of innate immunity. But still remain unresolved several questions before they become a new therapeutic agent against bacterial infections

Basic Concepts.

Mechanism Zipper: the microorganism contacts and adheres to the cell through the binding of a protein surface bacteria with its receptor on the cell surface (transmembrane protein adhesion). The cell then emits pseudopods modification of the cytoskeleton and encloses the bacteria in a vacuole. This mechanism is used by bacteria of the genus Yersinia and Listeria mechanism.

Trigger Bacteria interacts directly with the cellular cytoskeleton injecting bacterial effectors through a specialized secretion system. These effectors produce a massive rearrangement of the cytoskeleton to wrap the bacteria.

Phagolysosome Organelle surrounded by a single membrane, formed by the fusion of a lysosome (vacuole containing hydrolytic enzymes) and a phagosome (vacuole containing particles).

REFERENCE

1. Hooper LV: Do symbiotic bacteria subvert host immunity? Nature Reviews 2009; 7: 267 - 264.
2. Walker DH Rickettsiae and rickettsial infections: the current state of *knowledge. Clin.Infect. Dis. 2007,* **45,** S39-S44.
3. Santic, M., Molmeret, M., Klose, KE & Abu Kwaik, Y. Francisella tularensis travels a novel, twisted road Within macrophages. Trends Microbiol. 2006; 14, 37 44.
4. Flannagan RS; Cosio G and Grinstein S .: Antimicrobial Mechanisms of phagocytes and bacterial evasion strategies. Nature Reviews Microbiology 2009; 7: 355 - 366.
5. Ray K; Marteyn B; Sansonetti PJ and Tang CM .: life of the inside: the intracellular lifestyle of citosolyc bacteria. Nature 2009; 7: 333 - 340.
6. Santic, M., Asare, R., Skrobonja, I., Jones, S. & Abu Kwaik, Y. Acquisition of the vacuolar ATPase proton pump and phagosome acidification are essential for escape of *Francisella tularensis* macrophage into the cytosol. *Infect. Immun.* **76,**2671-2677 (2008).
7. Shaughnessy, LM, Hoppe, AD, Christensen, JA & Swanson, JA Membrane perforations inhibit lysosome fusion by altering pH and calcium in *Listeria* vacuoles monocytogenes. *Cell. Microbiol.* **8,**781-792 (2006).

Chapter 3

Antimicrobial Resistance

The development of effective antimicrobial agents has been one of the greatest achievements of modern science. However, the emergence of resistant organisms, has come to counteract all antimicrobials developed here, often limiting their usefulness.

The antimicrobial resistance has now become the silent epidemic of the XXI century and, until now, there has I could be stopped.a non-genetic origin of this resistance is known, as shown by some bacteria, in certain circumstances are inactive and do not multiply. This happens, for example, mycobacteria, which often survive in tissues for years after infection, braking by host defense mechanisms, which does not propagated and therefore cannot be eradicated but if the patient's cellular immunity is suppressed, they become vulnerable, sensitive to these drugs. However, this source of resistance is less significant. The further development of bacterial resistance to antimicrobials has been accelerated by mass production of this type of drug that started after 1940.

It is ironic and paradoxical that antimicrobial agents the best available so far for the treatment of infections, are also the most important agents of selection and spread of resistant bacteria.

Many experts agree that at least half of the human use of antimicrobials, whether in the community and in hospitals, it is unnecessary and inappropriate . Even better results have been confirmed in some parts of the world, although the actual extent of the problem remains unknown.

We are paying the concept that antibiotics have been a "miracle" ... The initial erroneous impression that after its discovery They consider them as "miracle drugs" is exacting a heavy price 1930s.;

ORIGIN OF Antimicrobial RESISTANCE

The sulfamídicos, who first Antibacterial who entered the trade in the They succeeded with its initial efficiency, extensive use in Japan in 1940, primarily in the treatment of bacillary dysentery (Shigella). However, 10 years later between 80-90%

of Shigella isolated in this country were resistant to sulfonamide. Chloramphenicol, streptomycin and tetracycline was then used widely and effectively; more resistant strains began to appear to these antimicrobials and even some multiresistant.

The use of penicillin as only drug set a precedent that this could be used for any infection and that was for almost 10 years. However, after that time in England begins to report the emergence of resistance to this drug and soon the world was shocked to realize that the same thing was happening all over the planet.

The Fleming himself warned in 1945 that the misuse of penicillin could lead to the selection and spread of mutant forms in the laboratory and correctly ruled that the situation could become worse when the drug could be obtained on a formula to be dispensed orally. Nobody paid attention to that warning then.

Soon after, between 60-70 years, the euphoria experienced by the emergence of penicillin began to decline with the growing resistance of germs to it, forcing the search for other antimicrobials allowed to address the problem created. What was happening?

Resistance plasmids

The first disturbing elements began to be observed in cases of patients infected by Escherichia coli in which multiple resistance was observed against antimicrobials. Known that this germ, opposite the selective pressure imposed by the use of antimicrobials, in this case the sulfonamide, spontaneously mutated and transferred strength characteristics to their offspring, developing drug-resistant mutants. (Chromosomal resistance)

In 1959 several investigations indicated that the transfer of this resistance, which required contact cell to cell without being mediated filterable agents such as phages or DNA was occurring independently of chromosomal transmissibility was born ... transferable concept extrachromosomal elements containing genes resistant which was called plasmid or factor R. (extrachromosomal Resistance)

In 1966 already 75% of strains of Shigella had multiple resistance to streptomycin and sulfonamide and of these, about 90% were able to transfer this resistance to susceptible organisms receiver, but ... how about transferring this resistance itself and others not?

He soon learned that there were several types of plasmids and that they used different mechanisms through which the transfer occurred and resistance The following definitions are

1. Plasmid:

Extrachromosomal genetic element that plays independently to the host chromosome

2. Plasmid Resistance:

A plasmid which carries genetic information for resistance to various antibiotics. Including the various mechanisms for transfer of resistance were identified:

- Plasmid Conjugation:
  A plasmid can start and lead the transfer
  unilateral of genetic material from a bacterium resistant to other sensitive, by binding two compounds to produce a third party or the union of two agencies to exchange its nuclear substance, though not are of the same gender.

- Plasmid Non conjugative:
  A plasmid alone cannot carry out the transfer of resistance by conjugation, however is performed by:

  - Transformation:
  The naked DNA of a cell passes from one species to another altering, therefore, its genotype. This can occur through laboratory manipulation

  - Transduction
  The genetic material is enclosed in a bacterial virus (bacteriophage) and transferred by the virus to other bacteria of the same plasmid species.

In general, it can be clearly defined although not usually encode functions essential for the bacterium, so are unnecessary for growth of the microorganism, they contain additional genetic information responsible for the appearance of new phenotypic properties in the bacterial cell (confer resistance, toxin production, containing genes capable of provide the bacteria's ability to metabolize certain substrates, etc.)

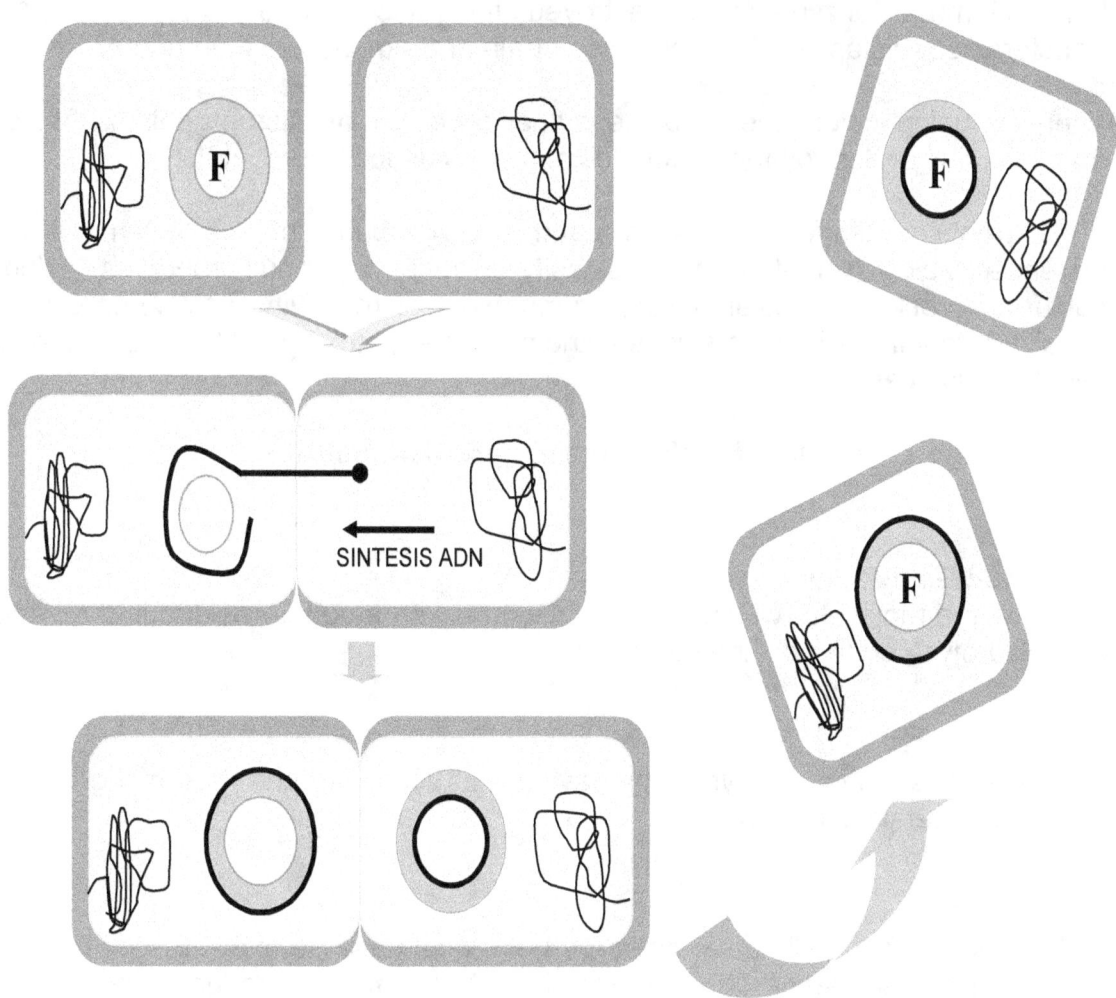

Mediated resistance mechanisms of plasmids

Not everything is explained further with this knowledge and the fact is that the R (resistance plasmids) factors expanded around the world.

Betalactamases

Japanese observers noted that despite the increasing emergence of resistance in the world of aminoglycosides (especially to kanamycin, neomycin and ampicillin) it was very rare in Japan, where infrequent use of these products led to correlate the use of antimicrobial and subsequent development of resistance.

Soon after it was found that there was resistance mediated by the presence of a beta-lactamase enzyme that destroyed the discovery of penicillin in 1965 transferable resistance to ampicillin in a strain of Salmonella typhimurium.

Then beginning to describe a group enzymes produced by microorganisms that were able to inhibit or destroy the antimicrobial agents used to combat them.

The current knowledge about diversity and wide distribution of beta-lactamases have increased rapidly. You attempted to classify response to various properties, including substrate profile, molecular weight, immunological reactivity with some antisera, sensitivity to various inhibitors, isoelectric properties, etc., but all these schemes are full of ambiguities.

Classification according betalactamases profilesubstrate

- ### Class A:
They have a molecular weight of about 29,000, with a serine residue in their active site. Hydrolyze preferably the penicillins.

- ### Class B
They are called metalloenzymes by having a structure around the Thiol group zinc required forbetalactamásica

- ### Class C
Included chromosomally determined by beta-lactamase genes of E. coli K-12 and also extended sequences homologous to beta-lactamase produced by Klebsiella chromosomally and Shigella. These enzymes are long protein with molecular weight of about 39,000 and possess a wide activity against cephalosporins. The tertiary structure that has this kind of betalactamases makes them very similar to the structure of the PFP (penicillin binding proteins) that can be confused with.

Class D
Included beta-lactamases that hydrolyze to oxacillin

A scheme that may be appropriate to some extent, the divided response:

- **Antimicrobial they attack:**
- penicillinase
- cephalosporinases
- Oxacilinasas
- Carbenicilinasas
- Carbapenemases

- Cefaminasas. etc.
- **A genetic information necessary for production:**
- plasmid
- Chromosomal
- **The type of training:**
- Permanent
- Temporary
- **A amino acid and nucleotide sequences:**
- Class A
- Class B
- Class C
- Class D
- **Al profile substrate and inhibition by clavulanic acid:**
- Broad spectrum
- spectrum spread

The arrangement of semisynthetic penicillins and derivatives Cephalosporins increasingly resistant to the effect of most beta-lactamases have partially improved the situation, but not resolved ... It seems that for every derivative created so far there are, at some level, one lactamase to hydrolyze them.

Beta-lactamases have continued and today are already described a huge number of

Main betalactamases

betalactamases	PL	Prevalence	Guest BACTERIA.
1 Wide range.			
HMS-1	5.2	Rare	Enterobacteriaceae
TEM-1	5.4	Very common	Enterobacteriaceae P. Aeruginosa H. V. Cholera influenzae N. gonorrhoeae
TLE-1	5.55	Rara	E. Coli
TEM-2	5.6	Joint	Enterobacteriaceae
CSF-1	5.85 or 6.5		
		Rara	P. aeruginosa
NPS-1	6.5		
TLE-2			K. Pneumoniae
LXA-1	6.7	Uncommon	Enterobacteriaceae
OHIO-1	7.0		E.Cloacae S. Marcensces
SHV-1 (PIT-2)	7.6	Joint	Enterobacteriaceae
ROB-1	8.1	Uncommon	H. Influenzae

			K.pneumoniae P.Multocida
2. Oxacilinasas.			
OXA-9	6.9	Rare	K. Pneumoniae
OXA-3	7.1	Uncommon	Enterobacteriaceae P. Aeruginosa
OXA-1	7.4	Common	
OXA-4	7.45	Rare	Enterobacteriaceae
OXA-8?	7.6		
OXA-5	7.62		P.aeruginosa
OXA-7	7.65		E. Coli
OXA-6	7.68		P aeruginosa
OXA-2	7	Common	Enterobacteriaceae P.aeruginosa.
3 Carbenicilinasas.			
CARB-4	4.3	Rare	P. Aeruginosa
SAR-1	4.9		V. Cholera
PSE-4. (CARB-1)	5.3	Uncommon	P.aeruginosa Enterobacteriaceae
BRO-1 BRO-2-3 BRO	multi-band (5.3-7.7)	Common	Bramahella
PSE-1. (CARB-2)	5.7		P.aeruginosa Enterobacteriaceae
CARB-3	5.75	Rara	P. Aeruginosa
CARB-5	6.3		A. Calcoaceitus
PSE-3	6.9	Uncommon	P.aeruginosa Enterobacteriaceae
N-29	6.9 (6.93)	Rarely	P. Mirabilis

betalactamases	PL	Prevalence	host
4.Extended spectrum. Class A of the related oximino-lactamase TEM, SHV, or OXA beta-lactamases (confer resistance to cefotaxime, ceftazidime and aztreonam)			
Derivatives TEM			
TEM-3-29 TEM	5.2-6.5	Present in nosocomial infections	K. Pneumoniae
TEM-42 TEM-43			Less common in other Enterobacteriaceae
TEM-46 TEM-67			

Derivatives SHV			
SHV-2-12 SHV	7.0-8.2	Present in nosocomial infections	K.pneumoniae Less common in other Enterobacteriaceae
TEM-30, TEM-40		only found in infections nosocomialin France and Spain	E. Coli
TEM-44 TEM-45			
Derivatives OXA			
OXA-11 OXA-14 OXA-16	6.1-8.0	insulation innosocomial Turkey	P.aeruginosa.

5 Other classes A oximino-lactamase unrelated to TEM, SHV, or OXA beta-lactamases.
Cefuroxime confer resistance to

CTX-M-2	5.5	insulation in Argentina	S. Typhimurium E. Coli V. Cholera
Toho-1	7.8	insulation in Japan	E. Coli
Toho-2?		Insulation in UTIs in Japan	
MEN-1 (CTX-M-1)	8.4	insulation in France and Germany	
CTX-M-April		insulation in ITU at a hospital in Poland	E. Coli C. Freundi
CTX-M-June		insulation in Russia	S.Typhimurium

Related with PER that confer resistance to Ceftibuten			
PER-1	5.4	Isolated in some hospitals in Turkey	P. Aeruginosa K.pneumoniae Acinetobacter
PER-2		isolates in Argentina	S. Typhimurium and some other Enterobacteriaceae that are not P. aeruginosa

betalactamases	PL	PREVALENCE	Host
6. bacteria.Class C Cefaminicinasas (confer resistance to cefoxitin or Cefotetan)			
MIR-1	8.4	Isolated in a hospital in Providence	K.pneumoniae
ACT-1	9.0	Isolated in nosocomial infections in New York City Hospital	E. Coli K.pneumoniae
BIL-1	8.8	Isolated in a burned child in Pakistan	E.coli
CMY-2	9.0	isolated from patients with UTI in Athens, Greece	K.pneumoniae C.freundi
SALT-1		Isolated on stools in Nigeria	S.Senftenberg
LAT-1	9.4	serious nosocomial infections in Greece	K. Pneumoniae
LAT-2	9.4, 9.1, 8.8		K. Pneumoniae E.coli E.Aerogenes
MOR-1?		S.enteritis	
RelatedFOX			
FOX-1	6.8 or 7.2	Isolated blood from patients in a hospital in Buenos Aires	K.pneumoniae
FOX-2	6.7	Isolated in ITU paraplegicof Guatemala	E.coli
FOX-3	7.25	vaginal insulation in Italy	oxytocaK-1
CMY	8.0	Isolated in Korea	K.pneumoniae
OX-1	8.9	Isolated in ITU in Nagoya, Japan	
Strangers			
CEP-1	8.0	rarely	P. mirabilis
7. Carbapenemases (confers resistance to imipenem or Meronemen) **metalloenzymes (Class B beta-lactamase)**			
IMP-1	9.0	Isolated in Japan	P. Aeruginosa S. Marcensces K. pneumoniae P. putida
unnamed			B. Fragilis
ARI-1	6.65	Isolated in blood of patients in Scotland	A.baumannii
ARI-2	7.1	isolated in Argentina,	Acinetobacter spp

		also found in Europe and Southeast Asia	

Antimicrobial resistance caused by these enzymes is one of the most serious and troubling problems of the present.

Since 1992 it has been pointing out that genes ESBLs some, previously restricted to sites of the chromosome, are transmitted between bacteria through plasmids. Plasmid-encoded beta-lactamases are a particular concern because of the possibility of increased bacterial resistance among different species of pathogens.

Against these inhibitory agents (IBL), lactam derivatives virtually no antibacterial activity, but capable of being detected by arose bacterial beta-lactamase inducing them to engage them and destroying itself inseparably both.

These inhibitors *"suicide"* as some have called the romantically, they managed to stop a little resistance but outside of that success, we can not say that we won the battle yet.

Transposons

Another important fact that added to these discoveries was the presence of factors R in normal untreated with antibiotics.

At the beginning of 1970 likely will be better clarified the mechanism for disseminating a particular genetic element between Plasmids, and indeed for their evolution. It was found that a DNA segment could translocate or transposing from one zone to another DNA itself; that is, they were able to "jump" from one plasmide to another, from plasmid to chromosome, and then again chromosome to plasmid.

This transposition mechanism appears to involve the inclusion of these "jumping genes" in a variety of possible locations without relying . general recombination function

well came the concept of transposon as defined genetic element that can translocate well as a genetic locus to another intact; ie DNA segment capable of moving from one position to another in the genome, or from the chromosomal DNA into a plasmid or vice versa recognized..

a new mechanism by which can transfer the resistance it is then transposition

Transposons were discovered by first in E. coli strains for the study of a class of highly polar mutations in the galactose and lactose operons. It was noted that the observed mutations simply could not be offset by base substitutions or mutagens exchange network, but only by cleavage of a DNA fragment.

So today many types of transposons are known, but generally, those found in Bacteria can be divided into three types:

1. Insertion sequences (IS):

These are the simplest. They are normal constituents of bacterial chromosomes and can be integrated into plasmids and phage genomes. Only carry the genetic information necessary for its own transfer (ie, the gene encoding the transposase). It is possible to detect whether your insertion leads to disruption or inactivation of genes, or modify the expression of adjacent genes. His appearance is as follows:

A B C D E F	tnp	F´E´D´C´B´A´

2. Complex transposons:

They are called R factors (high medical interest as they are the most common cause of active antimicrobial resistance). They are carried by conjugative plasmids. They have two functionally distinct parts: the resistance transfer factor and the transposon containing the genes for various types of drug resistance. Transposons carried by conjugative plasmids can be divided into two categories or generational types:

• The **type I** central region containing a selective carrying genes, for example, antimicrobial resistance, flanked on both sides by two identical elements or SI almost identical

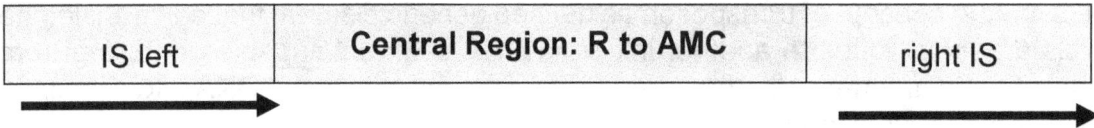

IS left	Central Region: R to AMC	right IS

• Type **II** transposons which are quite large and are not considered compounds, because they do not require the presence of SI modules for transposition. Instead, each member of these transposons is joined by two short repeats of 30 to 40 base pairs in length. Its central region contains 3 genes. One encoding resistance to AMC, the other two genes encode proteins involved in the transposition process. They just transposonan by satellite replicative

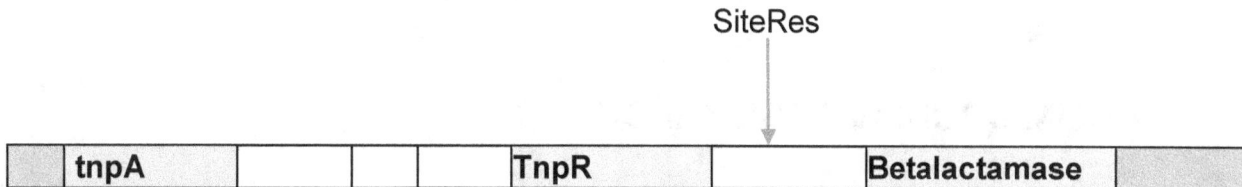

3. Phage Transpositivos:

Also known as transposons associated phages. They use transposition as normal playback mode integrated into the host genome after infection. Prophage insertion generally inactivates the bacterial gene in which it is inserted, disrupting the coding sequence and terminate transcription. Distal can also inactivate genes in the same plasmid operon; transposon. The existence implies that factors can increase their resistance R capturing genes of various origins as phage, chromosomes and other and then disseminate.

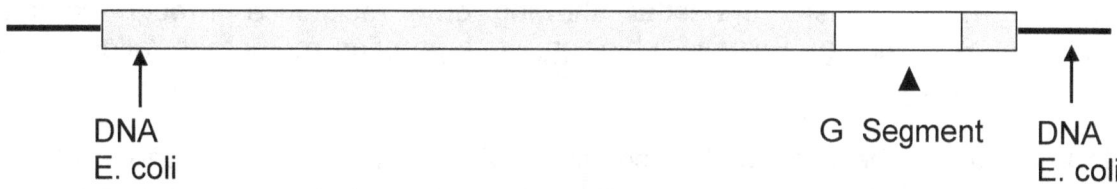

The impact of resistance traslocable quickly put in doubt, some of the therapeutic principles more firmly established in Pediatrics and Venereology, especially those related to treatment with Ampicillin of meningitis caused by H. influenzae and treatment with Neisseria gonorrhoeae Penicillin respectively

Ampicillin was for more than 10 years the drug of choice in Haemophilus meningoencephalitis; however, this germ acquired resistance to this drug from the existing pool of resistance among enteric gram-negative bacilli, forcing them to start using Chloramphenicol, already today also suffers increasing this resistance so they have begun to use third-generation cephalosporins in the treatment of this entity.

The origin of plasmids or resistance R factors is not well known. Antimicrobial mass production began after 1940 has been very important to select and disseminate R factors, and may have accelerated evolution, but it is almost certainly not created.

(Remember that all true antimicrobials are produced by microorganisms, especially Actinomycetaes, so very likely that they exist on earth since time immemorial).

The one fact there is no doubt is that the main factor responsible for the phenomenon of resistance Bacterial is the use and misuse of antimicrobials.

ANTIMICROBIAL RESISTANCE

Antimicrobial, although they have saved and improved more lives than any other kind of medicine, have led to its use, the largest intervention on the genetics of bacterial populations known so far.

It is known that some antimicrobials may have some natural resistance to certain antibiotics. . However, it is more common that this resistance is acquired

As we stated earlier, not all provoke resistance plasmids or not all R factors are mediated by the same mechanism; but even so we can say that all resistance is mediated by plasmids. In some cases, the resistance is very important mediated chromosomally identical to plasmid-mediated mechanisms. Pathogens acquire this resistance by incorporating a factor in their genes that makes the antimicrobial ineffective, and transmit that resistance to their offspring via plasmids or transposons. Thus everything is ready so that after multiple contacts between the antimicrobial and the microorganism, the latter showing drug resistance through complex mechanisms including:. Enzyme inhibition, waterproofing membrane, altering wall precursors, etc.

No but knowing these general mechanisms of resistance is not much help to the doctor, except in theory. It is necessary to interpret the same in each antimicrobial group to be known as pathogens become resistant to them.

There are many basic mechanisms from which the antimicrobial offer antimicrobial

1. Failure to penetration of the antimicrobial through outer membrane

Such is the case of the resistance observed in Gram negative germs to penicillin. In these cases the outer membrane of the same acts as a very efficient barrier penetration antimicrobial due to the presence of compounds for hydrocarbon molecules lipopolysaccharide preventing entry of the drug into the bacterial cell.

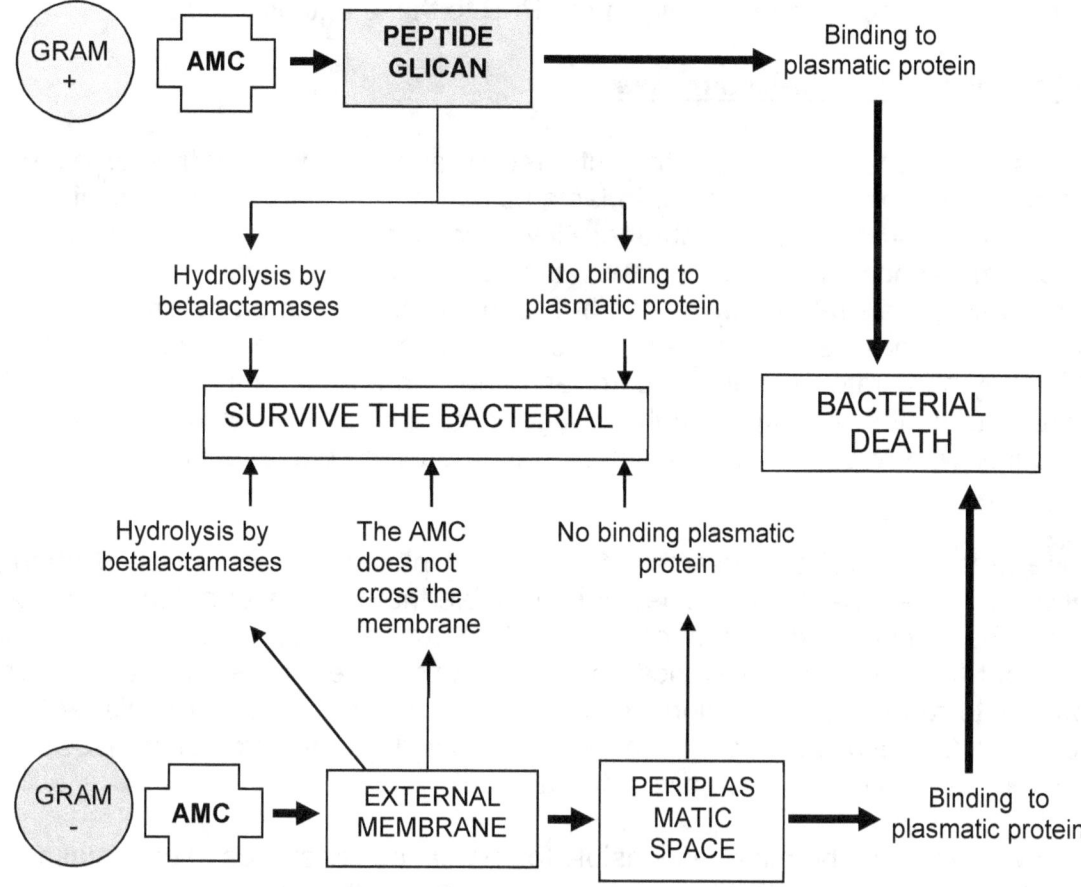

Mechanisms of bacterial resistance to antimicrobial acting on cell wall

Addition, this penetration of lactams requires mandatory passage of drug through porins existing channels (pores) in the outer membrane. Mutation of porin protein can cause the body also becomes resistant to these drugs. An example of this type of resistance mechanism shown in Pseudomonas aeruginosa to imipenem.

2. Failure of the bonding of the antimicrobial to the target site

In Gram negative bacteria to beta-lactam resistance is related to a decrease in the affinity of penicillin binding proteins (PFP) or these antimicrobials by a change in the amount of PFP produced by these bacteria. This mechanism is responsible for the resistance of staphylococci to oxacillin and penicillin resistance in Streptococcus pneumoniae.

Neisseria gonorrhoeae, Neisseria meningitidis, Haemophilus influenzae and Streptococcus pneumoniae are examples of seeds that have become resistant to many beta-lactam incorporate in their plasmids carrying resistance genes information to decrease the affinity of the PFP to these antimicrobials.

3. <u>Hydrolysis by beta-lactamases</u>

The particular characteristics of the outer membrane of Gram negative force already explained previously, as we said, to lactams can only access the interior of the cell through the pores of the membrane. However, once achieved penetration to the periplasmic space have to contend with the hydrolyzing beta-lactamase enzymes, in these cases, are strategically placed between the outer membrane and the PFP. In this position, these enzymes can destroy the antimicrobial molecules sequentially while they penetrate through the pore, as if they were abundant sniper ammunition pointing to white passing through a single entry point. This occurs, for example, compared with Ampicillin in strains of E. coli producing beta-lactamase.

Since these potent beta-lactamases present in plasmids and can be exchanged between different bacterial species, it is possible that the use of antimicrobial beta-lactam be constrained in the not too distant future. This becomes even more important to define this resistance as induced or transient type, that is, opposite it appears to repetitive and prolonged use of these types of antimicrobials (selective pressure). Cephalosporins are the most exposed to the expression of drug resistance due to increased use that are given, for its great.

Then we can say The main responsible for increased resistance to cephalosporins, even the most recent outings market are its magnificent broad-spectrum antimicrobial properties, which has currently used, with increasing frequency to treat any infection that does not have a "normal" evolution but it is solvable with other antimicrobial less powerful.

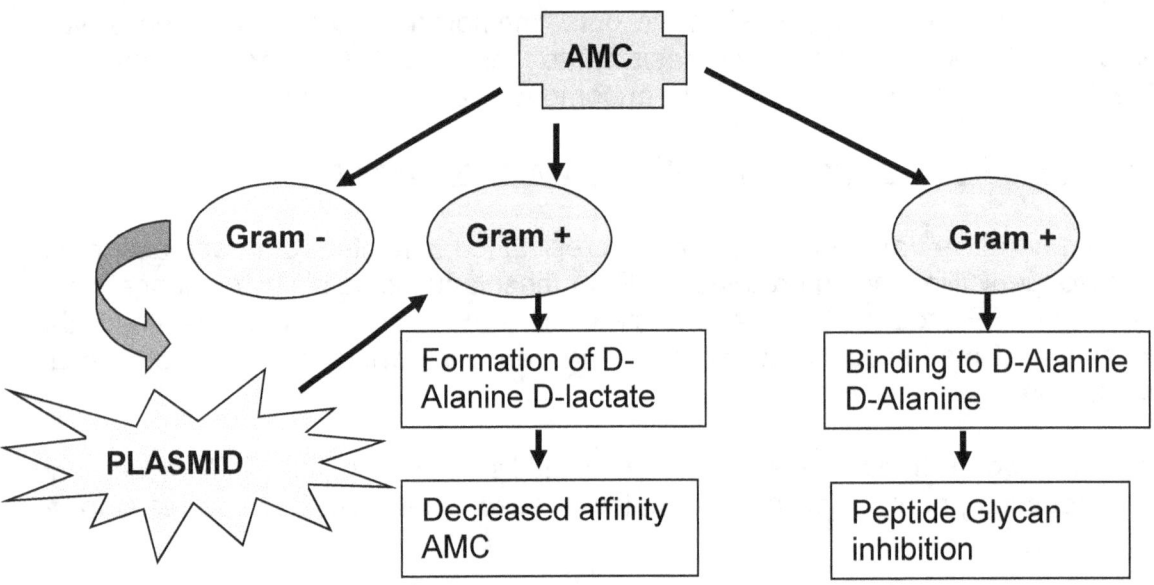

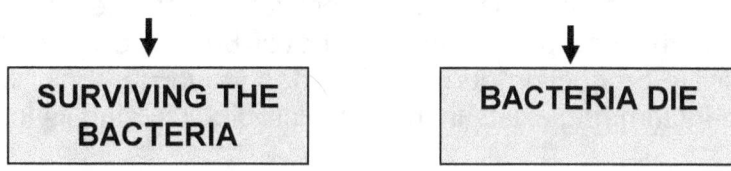

| SURVIVING THE BACTERIA | BACTERIA DIE |

Mechanism of bacterial resistance to Vancomycin

This antibiotic resistance is produced by changes in the target site of drug (presence of D-lactate instead of D-alanine) that alters the terminal or side chain of a protein production interfere with the binding of the antimicrobial to the target site.

In 1999 it was said that the vancomycin resistance among Gram-positive bacteria was not common. In 2001 and outbreaks of Staphylococcus epidermidis and Staphylococcus aureus resistant to this antibiotic, as well as an increase of the resistance into other Gram-positive species that were previously sensitive reported.

This progressive and rapid proliferation of resistance between positive Gram this antimicrobial has forced to take strict measures to control its use, especially in hospital settings where were plasmids isolated in an hour transmitted resistance gene to other species of bacteria present in the environment.

4. <u>Anti-microbial inactivation by destroying or the</u> <u>modification thereof</u>

Examples of this mechanism are the beta-lactamase and aminoglycoside inactivating enzymes. Other examples of this mechanism are: The constitutive production of chloramphenicol acetyltransferase (CAT-Asa) mediated resistance plasmids or chromosomally then causes mutants with higher resistance values chromosomally.

Even this ratio Asa CAT-mediated and mediated plásmides can sometimes intertwined by recombination or transposition modifications..

In the case of aminoglycosides described three plasmids mediated enzymatic

- phosphorylation of hydroxyl groups (-OH) with ATP as phosphate donor
- acetylation of amino groups (- NH2) with acetyl CoA as acetyl donor.
- Adenylation hydroxyl groups cyclase ATP as donor.

Such modifications often result resistance enzymes producing bacteria to the drug. Also in this group it is known that over 80% of S. aureus in the US are resistant to penicillin production due to plásmides inducible penicillinase which hydrolyzes the beta-lactam ring exists in the antimicrobial, causing its inactivation.

5. Decreased permeability as preventing access to White

Can be of two types:

•   **Natural** As is known beta-lactam basically exert their antibacterial effect by inhibiting the transpeptidase, thus, inhibit the synthesis of peptide glycan layer of the cell wall. Remembering that Gram negative bacilli have this layer between an outer shell containing lipopolysaccharides and proteins and a cytoplasmic inner membrane phospholipid we can deduce that alongside these transpeptidases wall, there are there other enzymes are also inhibited by beta-lactams.

Now However, to achieve any of these proteins and exert their action, these antimicrobials have to traverse the outer membrane of the cell envelope that is known is capable of preventing penetration of several substances, including penicillins.

This natural barrier is important, not only because it explains the absolute or relative resistance to penicillin having Gram negative bacilli but also because it increases the resistance of the beta-lactamase producers controlling the rate at which these antimicrobials are available to such enzymes.

Another case of natural barrier to the permeability, is possessed by for Aminoglycosides Enterococci.

In clinical these germs are killed by much lower concentrations of aminoglycosides which are able to inhibit them in vitro synergistically when combined with an agent that interferes with cell wall synthesis. The mechanism of this synergy has shown that includes an increased uptake and accumulation of the drug by the bacteria, thus allowing passing through what would otherwise be a very effective permeability barrier·.

        Acquired factors mediated Tetracycline resistance in Gram negative rods R and inducible S. aureus includes a decreased uptake of the drug.

Reports the existence of a new protein in E. coli membranes containing R factor for Tetracyclines in minicells incubated in the presence of the antimicrobial suggests that this resistance can include inducible synthesis of a new protein that acts on the cell membrane decreasing or increasing the penetration of the antimicrobial output.

6. Alteration of the target site of the antimicrobial

In these cases they bring different variants resistance may occur:

a) Increased concentration of competitive substances: As with sulfamídicos that exert their action by establishing competition with PABA for dihydropteroate synthase enzyme involved in the first step of the synthesis of folic acid. There are strains of S. aureus that are resistant to these

Antimicrobials because they produce twenty times more sensitive than their counterparts PABA, and therefore exceed competitive inhibition of these drugs.

b) Synthesis of a tough white area: In many bacteria ribosomal when exposed in vitro or in vivo changes occur streptomycin. This resistance results from the change of a single amino acid in a protein of the 30s ribosomal subunit, which normally binds the drug. This prevents the binding with consequent inhibition of protein synthesis and misreading of the genetic code. Other times the macrolide resistance ribosomal dependent rRNA alteration, specifically a methylation Nucleotide sequence of ribosomal 23s decreasing fixing these antimicrobial 50s ribosome as in S. aureus. Also resistant white area can occur by a decrease in affinity dihydropteroate synthetase, but unchanged affinity to the PABA; which means that the ability of drugs as Sulfas to serve as a competing product is disturbed as suggested by studies in Pneumococcus, gonococci and meningococci.

c) Synthesis of alternative white areas: Studies have shown that R factors may cause an alternative synthesis enzyme that prevents the inhibitory action of a drug on chromosomal enzyme. Several species of Gram negative bacteria with R factors for sulfamídicos have two dihydropteroate synthetase enzymes easily separated by their physical properties. A plasmid is measured, so it resists the in vitro inhibitory effects on the synthesis of folic acid; another is a "Wild" chromosomally mediated and still retains its susceptibility to these inhibitory effects.

From the above, it clearly deduce that are many different mechanisms by virtue of which the bacteria can resist the action of antimicrobials. In some cases they represent existing processes in nature. The emergence of resistant organisms in many, perhaps most, represents the final result of selective pressure by the extensive use of antimicrobials.

It is proved that today the only practical solution to the problem of bacterial resistance is to control the indiscriminate use of antimicrobials.

7. Efflux pumps.

This mechanism carries the antimicrobial from inside the bacteria unchanged but without antimicrobial action. There are multidrug efflux pumps in the cell wall that allow the expulsion of antimicrobials. The genes involved are MEF (respiratory syncytial), Nora (S. aureus) and Mex (Pseudomonas aeruginosa). These genes explain the resistance to macrolides and fluoroquinolones these pathogens. To combat this type of resistance are being studied the association of inhibitors of efflux pumps with the antimicrobial.

Antimicrobial resistance

World antimicrobials currently used in 20% of cases treated as outpatients and 40% of patients who require hospitalization, most of which are prescribed, they are not necessary or are administered in inappropriate doses. Similarly, too often they are given antimicrobials for treatment of minor infections or produced by viruses such as common cold.

In agriculture, these substances are also present, forming part of herbicides and other products widely used in the same. In livestock, food industry, etc. also they play a role. For example, veterinary sometimes uses them indiscriminately; both to prevent or treat diseases, as for growth of animal mass. Its waste can be obtained through meat, milk and its derivatives or other products intended for human consumption, representing a potential danger to our health and fostering unlimited resistance to them.

All these situations have led to significant changes in some concepts: To say today that microorganisms are the cause of infections is inadequate and incomplete; it is ignored in this way influence the recipient; in this case the man, the surrounding environment, and social and physical environment in which we evolved. It is worth recalling the close relationship between microorganism, host and antimicrobial. In this trilogy, the former have developed an extraordinary capacity to resist destruction by creating mechanisms to inhibit or destroy the antimicrobial.

So much so that, in studies, it has been found that the S. pneumoniae in 6 years progressively increased resistance to penicillin and rose by 32% intermediate susceptibility. But most alarming is what is happening at the community level with the same drug resistance obtained where carriers 1 year, is already 61.4%.

In the case of H. influenzae type b (Hib), before applying the vaccine in Cuba he represented the etiologic agent of more than 33% of bacterial meningitis. In 1999, after application of the vaccine, morbidity declined by 59%, but the germ has been showing high strength, inclusive, and drugs such as ceftriaxone and 40% of beta-lactam strains exhibit activity. Non capsulated strains of this bacteria are observed in children carriers with a higher strength than for capsulated strains tetracycline and chloramphenicol.

Shigella is presenting a statistically significant increase in resistance to nalidixic acid, used as drug of choice to combat it. Gentamicin, this germ shows a resistance of 2.5% and the rest of the tested drugs did not observe changes in their pattern of resistance.

Other research shows that the S. Typhi in our country has shown resistance to chloramphenicol 21-22%, 41-46% of the trimethoprim, from 12% to nalidixic acid and has since 1997 consistently increasing their resistance to ampicillin. Also today N. meningitidis type b is resistant to penicillin of 88.9%.

While it is true that the resistance patterns of our country with other countries, are very different, because even the crisis does not affect us in the same amount as is already affecting other places, we are not exempt from the phenomenon follow progressing and we meet soon face an impasse.

It is shown that the adaptive response of germs respond to selective pressure imposed on them by the antimicrobial and there is no doubt that so far, the response has been more rapid, efficient and robust than the manipulations performed by man in the chemical structure antimicrobial molecules for new products capable of combat.

REFERENCE

- Infectología Pediátrica. Resistencia de los betalactámicos a los gérmenes Gram positivos. Vol. IV Clin Med Norteam, 1997.

- Murray PR Medical microbiology. 4ta ed. Ed. Mosby. Vol. 4: 195-395, 2002.

- Goodman and Bilman. Las bases farmacológicas de la terapéutica. Vol II 9 ed (2): 1996.

- Monthly. Over us antibiotic. Prescribing referentes. Ed. Sales-Sataff. 188-208, 2005.

- Jawetz E et al. Microbiología médica. 15ta ed. México, DF Ed. El Manual Moderno SA, 1996.

- Rudolph H. Antibacterial therapy. 20th ed. Ed. Appleton and Lange. 444, 1996.

- Llop H. A, Valdés-Dapena V. Ma. M. Microbiología y Parasitología médicas Ed. Ecimed. Tomo I. 81-99, 2001.

- Alarma por el aumento de la resistencia bacteriana. Información para el desarrollo de la salud en América. Ed. El Hospital (issn) Vol. 6 (4): 2005.

- Llop HA et al. Resistencia a los antimicrobianos y vigilancia microbiológica en Cuba. En: Resistencia antimicrobiana en las Américas: Magnitud del problema y su contención. Ed. OPS/HCP/HCT/163/2000; 116-123.

- Neu HC The crisis of antibiotic resistance. Science 1992;257:1064-1073.

- Ramírez MM, Marrero M, Monté RJ, et al. Resistencia a la Ampicilina mediada por plásmidos R en cepas de Shigella flexneri. Rev Cub Med Trop 1994;46:148-151.

- Grady R. Pediatr Infect Dis J. 22,1128,2003.

- Payen S, Serreau R, Munck A, et al. Antimicrob Agents. Chemother, 47, 3170, 2003.

- Huy G, D'haene K, Collard JM, Swings J. Appl Environ Microbiol, 70, 1555, 2004.

Chapter 4

Multidrug resistant microorganisms

Resistant multidrug microorganisms (MMDR) have important implications for infection control, but despite the danger to health institutions and the community, since it has proved its spread from centers Community health to the environment; the problem has not been well focused and has received limited attention, perhaps because many professionals portend a speedy arrest of the problem but the reality is quite daunting to be seen exponential growth of the phenomenon of antimicrobial resistance by microorganisms.

The experience on these organisms it has provided the necessary information to clarify the routes of transmission and effective prevention and control measures. Although initially linked and restricted to hospitals, the emergence and transmission of MMDR today affects all health institutions, dedicated to long-term care of people and community centers. The severity and extent of disease caused by these organisms vary according to the affected populations and the institutions where they are isolated. Regarding these institutions they vary widely in their physical structure and functional characteristics. As a result, the approach to the prevention and control of these pathogens need to be adapted to the specific needs of each population and institution.

The prevention and control of MMDR is a global priority it needs, urgently, governments, institutions own health or companies in the health sector, to assume the problem responsibly.administrations

Health and institutions should ensure that strategies are implemented properly and in accordance with the rules; regularly evaluate their effectiveness and adjust to achieve a substantial reduction in the incidence of these organisms.

To make sustainable prevention and control MMDR requires updates, directives and circulars administrative and scientific. Professionals and staff working in the health sector are more receptive and more adhere to the recommendations for prevention and infection control when there are organizational directives.

The following article provides guidance for the implementation of strategies and practices . MMDR prevention

Definition

MMDR resistant organisms are more than one group of antimicrobials.

Although certain MMDR name describes the resistance to a single agent (eg MRSA.), these pathogens are frequently resistant to most available and thus require special attention in health institutions. Of particular interest are MRSA, VRE and BEGN strains, including producers included ß - lactamases of extended spectrum (ESBL) and others that are resistant to several groups of antimicrobial agents. Just to mention some examples include: E. coli, Klebsiella pneumoniae and Acinetobacter baumannii resistant to all antibiotics except imipenem or all microorganisms and as Stenothrophomonas maltophilia, Burkhordelia cepacea and Raestonea picketti that are intrinsically resistant to all antimicrobials extended spectrum. In some centers for the care of chronic patients or without subsidiary protection, there are germs that have become epidemiological importance, as is the case of multidrug resistant pneumoniea Streptocccus; they are resistant to penicillins, macrolides and quinolones; S. aureus strains with reduced susceptibility or resistance to vancomycin (VISA and VRSA).

Clinical significance of multidrug-resistant microorganisms.

MMDR infections have similar infections caused by susceptible microorganisms clinical expression. However, treatment options for patients with infections MMDR are extremely limited. Only offered as vancomycin therapeutic effectiveness and safety against potentially lethal MRSA infections shortly after the infections were resistant to vancomycin (VRE). And although today it is available in the international market of new antibiotics to treat infections MRSA and VRE; resistance to each of these new agents emerge in different isolates of clinical samples. Likewise, treatment options are also limited to infections caused by ESBL-producing BEGN.

Infections caused by these organisms have implicit prolonged hospital stays with increasing costs and mortality. Vancomycin resistance is a predictor of mortality in bacteremia by Enterococcus. Meanwhile, MRSA colonized patients develop infections more often symptomatic with increased mortality occur primarily when bacteremia and infections of the surgical wound. This outcome may be due to a delay in prescribing vancomycin decreased susceptibility to vancomycin or persistent bacteremia associated with intrinsic characteristics of certain strains of MRSA.

Epidemiology

The prevalence varies widely from one geographical area to another, in time and Hospital. The type of care I provided also influences the prevalence. Multidrug resistance is higher in hospitals with intensive care, cardiovascular and transplant than those who do not have these special services units. Likewise, the prevalence of TB is higher in large hospitals VRE.; in 2000 found that 4% of patients were colonized with MRSA or 10. 2% were colonized by ESBL producers BEGN. Whether the evidence suggests that MDR is higher in adult hospitals, this requires similar prevention and control efforts in pediatric institutions.

In recent years the prevalence of MMDR in hospitals and medical centers has increased exponentially in most countries. In the United States, at the beginning of the 90s, MRSA accounted for 20 to 25% of S. aureus isolated from hospitalized patients; MRSA in 2003 reached 59.5%.A similar pattern of increase in multidrug resistance has been observed for Enterococcus, K. pneumoniae, P. aeruginosa and E. coli. In the hospital where we work a similar phenomenon has occurred MRSA observed a prevalence of 55.6%. The E. coli germ that until less than a decade showed excellent susceptibility patterns to most antibiotics ß- lactams and trimethoprim - sulfamethoxazole; in 2010, it showed high levels of resistance to penicillins, cephalosporins and carbapenems, showing the circulation of ESBL producing strains. Similarly, it has happened in the germs isolated from patients with nosocomial infections. The most alarming is the isolation of resistant to most antimicrobials BEGN available for treatment.

Bacterial resistance.

Through selection and exchange of genetic resistance elements, antimicrobial polifarmacoresistence promote the emergence of bacterial strains is reduced proliferation microorganisms of the administered drug sensitive normal human flora, but resistant strains persist and may become endemic to the hospital. The widespread use of antibiotics for treatment or prophylaxis is the main determinant of resistance. Prescription, often indiscriminate, antimicrobial favors the emergence of resistant and multiresistant bacteria, which have spread exponentially in health institutions. Today many strains of pneumococcus, Staphylococcus, Enterococcus and Bacillus tuberculosis are resistant to most or all of the antibiotics were once effective treatment.

In many hospitals are prevalent Klesiellas and multidrug resistant Pseudomonas. This issue is of critical importance vital in countries developing, which may not have the second-line antibiotics, more expensive or, if available, its price is unavailable.

Why MMDR are a health problems public?

1. Exponential increase in bacterial resistance to newer and broad spectrum antimicrobial.

2. Emergency and emergency re microorganisms.
3. A greater number of people live in overcrowded conditions.
4. Increased frequency of immune (age, disease, malnutrition, treatments) deficiency.
5. The development of bacterial resistance is inversely proportional to the discovery of new antimicrobial agents.
6. Increased morbidity and mortality.
7. Great economic impact. The global economic crisis has become more expensive costs of raw materials and therefore the production and market prices; forcing governments to disburse large sums of money that lead to a rise in health.

People are at the center of the phenomenon.

a. As main reservoir and source of microorganisms
b. As a main transmitter, notably during treatment.
C. Receptor as microorganisms, which become a new reservoir.

Fig. 4.1 pathogenesis of infections MMDR

The person in the center of phenomenon

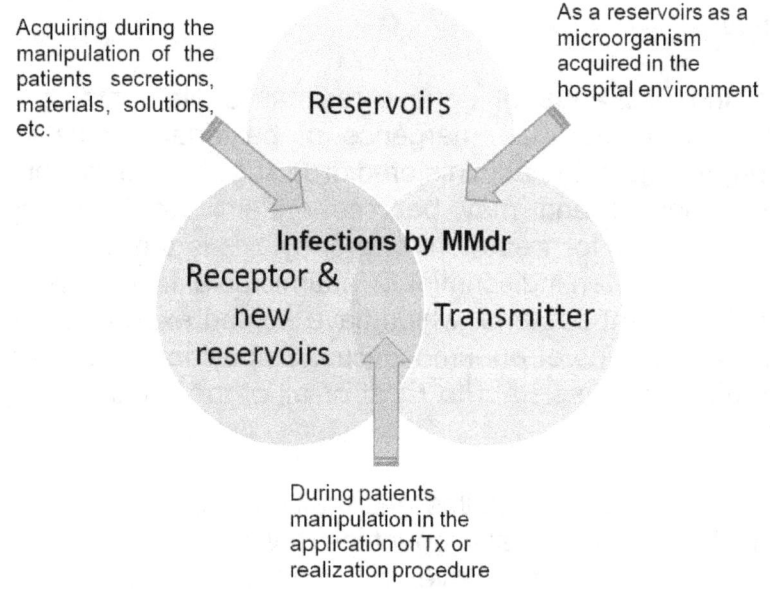

Fig. 4.2 Monitoring of MMDR is a circular process.

The microorganism surveillance is:

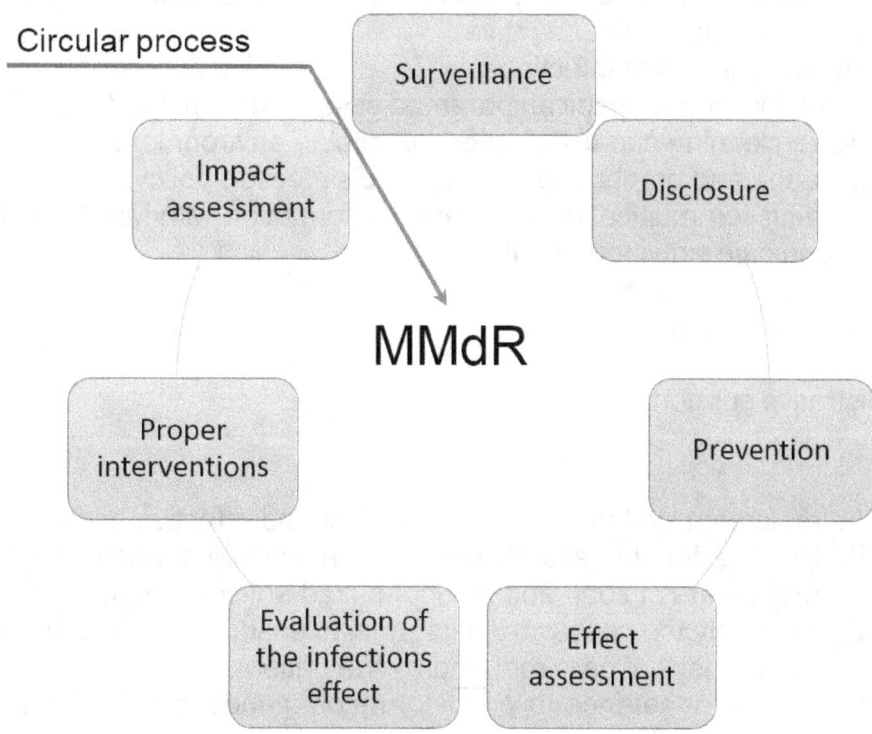

Prevention and control.

Preventing Infections.

Preventing infections of MMDR be reduced in health centers. Prevention of antimicrobial resistance depends on appropriate guidelines of good clinical practice, which should be incorporated into the care of all patients. These include optimal care of vascular and urinary catheters, prevention of infections of the lower respiratory tract in patients ventilated or tracheostomy, etiological diagnosis and appropriate selection and judicious use of antimicrobials.

Therefore control MMDR includes four basic strategies.

1. Prevention of infection.
2. Diagnosis and timely, early and appropriate treatment.
3. Prudent use of antimicrobials.
4. Transmission prevention.

Prevention and control of transmission MMDR.

a) Handwashing-.

b) Use of barriers to the contact (gloves, masks naso buco and lab coats) unless the cultures are negative
c) Active surveillance of infections
d) Health education to medical, paramedical , service, patients and families.
e) Increase cleaning and disinfection hospitable environment. Knowledge and proper use of hospital disinfection policy.
f) Improving communication and patient information with MMDR within and between care providers health.

Interventions for control.

a) Administrative support.

A. Implement systems to ensure a quick and effective communication.
B. Provide for the establishment of a sufficient number of sinks and dispensers of soap and alcohol-based antiseptic solutions.
C. Keep only the necessary personnel to ensure optimal care according to the intensity of care required by the patient.
D. Monitor adherence to practical recommendations for infection control studies.

b) Education: to disseminate results of microbiological graduate planning activities, with updated local and national epidemiological situation information.

c) Judicious use of antimicrobials and audit the use of the same, evaluating adherence to practice guidelines for diagnosis and treatment in force in the institution.

d) Monitoring MMDR

A. MMDR screening of cultures (susceptibility).
B. Appropriate use of antimicrobials in multidrug resistant strains and to prevent the emergence of MMDR.

I. The use of any antibiotic should be justified based on clinical diagnosis and known or anticipated infectious microorganisms.

II. Getting appropriate bacteriological examination before starting the antimicrobial therapy & clinical samples.

III. Knowing the patterns of sensitivity, tolerance and cost.

IV. Antimicrobial treatment in combination and correct dosage in sepsis and serious or potentially serious infections that may endanger the patient's life.

V. Antimicrobial monotherapy and reduced spectrum: mild infections; in moderate infections when the causative agent is known.

VI. Restrict the use of certain antibiotics.

REFERENCES

1. RJ Curtis, et al .: Intensive care quality improvement: a how-to guide for the interdisciplinary team. *Crit Care Med 2006;* 211-218

2..Siegel JD; Rhinehart E; Jackson M; Chiarello L and the healthcare infection monitoring advisory committee: management of multidrug - resistant organisms in healthcare setting,2006. http://www.cdc.gov/drugresistance/healthcare/

3..March Jabeen Kausar; Zafar Afia; Rumina Hasan: Frequency and sensitivity patterns of extended spectrum beta lactamase producing isolates in tertiary care hospital laboratory of Pakistan. J Pak Med Assoc. 2005; 55: 436 - 439.

4. Berriel - Cass D; Adkins F; Jones P; Fakih M .: Eliminating nosocomial infections at Ascension Health. J. Quality Patient Safety 2006; 32 (11): 612 - 620.

5. S. Shakil, SZ Ali, M. Akram, SM Ali, and AU Khana .: Risk Factors for Extended-Spectrum b-lactamase Producing Escherichia coli and Klebsiella pneumoniae Acquisition in a Neonatal Intensive Care Unit J Tropical Pediat 2010.;56 (2): 90 - 96.

6. Crivaro V, Bagattini M, Salza MF, et al. Risk factors for extended-spectrum beta-lactamase-producing Klebsiella pneumoniae and Serratia marcescens acquisition in a neonatal intensive care unit. J Hosp Infect 2007; 67: 135-41.

7. Bizzarro MJ Gallagher PG. Antibiotic-resistant organisms in the neonatal intensive care unit. Semin Perinatol 2007; 31: 26-32 Diseases..

Chapter 5

LABORATORY Microbiology and

Infectious Diseases

The realization of a group of additional tests on the patient in an infectious disease is suspected, provides considerable support to healthcare and allows, among other things, identify the causal agent and impose treatment Antimicrobial appropriate for its eradication.

By all it is known that antimicrobial agents, in recent decades, have radically altered the millennial struggle between the host and the invading agent, implying a different mode of attack on the pathogen, which joins alterations that this produces the pH, temperature and other own defensive measures the host.

The laboratory then allows the use of techniques that not only isolate, identify or cultivate pathogenic microorganisms, but also report on the susceptibility of the same against antimicrobial drugs that are used to fight and also make determinations schemes sensitivity and resistance to the drugs.

This has created a new era in drug treatment, which are seen increasingly details of the clinical pharmacology. The importance of laboratory tests continues to increase. Lately have been perfected many techniques that have required large financial investments but, in return, have provided the fruit of numerous data and information useful.

How can the doctor get the most out of this assistance, increasing, the lab gives?

Simply must be aware of the diagnostic methods that can be used to illuminate the path of healing.

The exogenous invaders cause disease in man are legion, ranging from virus, to Vermes and taenias really sizable. Some pathological processes can be correlated to some extent with the characteristics of the causative organism. This kind of knowledge is interesting and useful to some extent, but cannot fully explain the clinical course of the illness of a particular patient, although we can consider some factors that determine the scope and nature of the bacterial disease.

The pathogen must achieve an ecological relationship with its host, so that it can ensure its continuity as a species that is to say; it must penetrate and multiply within the host immediately leave to penetrate other or be able to survive independently.

Man has used the techniques of sanitation, antisepsis and sterilization to try to prevent the entry into the body of these and its transmission to other hosts. Antimicrobial agents, meanwhile, are trying to prevent the growth of microorganisms by preventing or correcting the harmful effects of this multiplication.

But pathogens are also facing these actions directed against them by their toxins (Endo and Exotoxins), developing or modifying resistance its features.

The diagnostic microbiology has paved the way for the identification of germs, their relationship to clinical situations, determining their patterns of sensitivity and drug resistance among others.

In general terms the identification of a significant pathogen required a clinically suitable material, appropriate bacteriological techniques are followed and that the resulting findings are interpreted in the light of general principles and individual circumstances be considered.

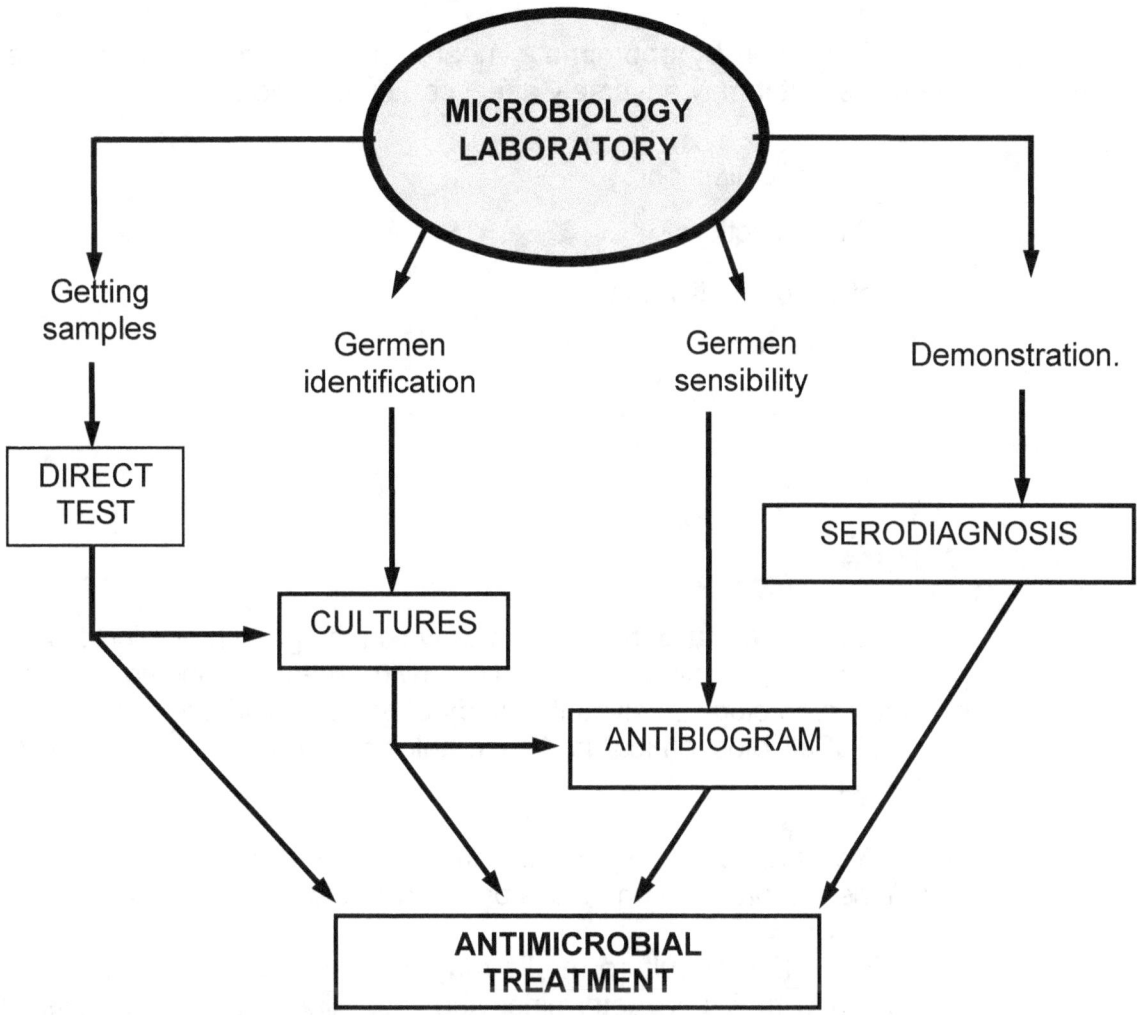

The microbiology laboratory to help treatment antimicrobial

Samples sent to the lab are intended get answers to several questions:

• Is there any microorganisms present there?

• If so, What are they?

• Are they related to the patient's illness?

• Are they pathogens?

- What therapeutic agents should be used in preference to combat?

Cultivation by appropriate means provides the most accurate these questions, but it may adversely affect certain situations.

- time of collection

- Site collection

- effect of medication

- Pollution

- Delayed culture

Culture

Is called **culture** the process by which the growth of microorganisms is promoted by providing appropriate environmental conditions. Almost all clinical microbiology involves the study of general cultivation techniques, and the use of all biochemical and morphological characteristics of pathogenic floraculture.

A culture containing only one kind of organism is known as **pure** which it comprises more than one class of organisms called **mixed** culture.

The different culture media may help or hinder the different types of bacteria and their use determines the most likely type of organism in the sample. To some extent, the origin of the samples microorganisms and suggests how the material should be used. However, in all cases, the more information available to the bacteriologist on the clinical problem, the more likely you are to achieve meaningful diagnostic results.

To study the properties of an organism is necessary not only to its isolation from naturally mixed microbial population, but also their maintenance and their offspring in isolated state, in an artificial environment in which the access of other microorganisms is prevented. For this purpose you can be used the following methods:

a) Seeding in plates:

The easiest way to obtain pure cultures of microorganisms form colonies on solid media, is performed by separating and immobilizing individual organisms on or in a solidified nutrient medium. Giving each cell there will grow an isolated colony whose transfer can be done easily. Planting in this medium is for flute and is performed using a sterile loop wire is inserted into the original suspension and then make a series of not overlapping, parallel striations on the plate. This method, generally satisfactory for isolation of bacteria and fungi

b) Dilution:

The simplest method of isolation liquid media widely used for insulating protozoa and consisting using a microorganism suspension, perform a serial dilution using a sterile medium and a large number of tubes inoculated with the culture medium, with aliquots of each of the serial dilutions. As a result, if a tube shows any subsequent growth, there is a high probability that this growth is the introduction of a single organism controlled.

c) Isolation microscopically

The microscope is the science that deals with the uses and applications Performing microscopes, which make very small particles may be perceived by the human eye. The scientific and technical development in this field has become milestones of progress in the knowledge of living organisms invisible to the human eye at first glance and achieved complete two main objectives: to form an enlarged image with the least possible amount of optical defects and achieve contrast to ensure the identification of germs, different structures, morphology, etc., using coloring substances. There are different types of microscopes and dyes used in the identification of microorganisms:

1. <u>Microscope:</u>
    - Simple Luminous
    - Luminous compound
    - phase contrast
    - darkfield
    - For fluorescence
    - Electronic
2. <u>Dyes:</u>
    - simple colorations
    - made colorations or differential
      - Gram stain
    - coloration of acid-fast microorganisms

- Ziehl-Neelsen
- Colouring Kinyoun

- negative stainings

- stainings to show structures of microorganisms:
  - Colouring of capsules
  - Colouring of flagella
  - Colouring spore
  - Colouring of metachromatic granules
  - Colouring core

- Other colorations

It is important that, even though count on these tools and techniques for the isolation and identification of germs, the time devoted to exposing the doctor in short clinical reference, the specific situation of the patient in the application the test can result in a faster and better culture performance.

In direct examination by microscopy, it is possible to detect the presence of products or infecting microorganism antigens by immunological methods and other cromatrographics. In direct examination of clinical samples and cytochemical study investigates the existence of microorganisms, inflammatory cells, proteins and glucose; providing a valuable diagnostic aid to provide the physician with a preliminary or definitive evidence of infected microorganism; facilitating the choice of appropriate and timely therapy.

The microscopic procedure performed most often is that of smears stained with Gram stain, useful in the etiological diagnosis of bacterial meningitis caused by Haemophilus influenzae, Neisseria meningitidis and Streptococcus pneumoniae. When the diagnosis of meningitis was premature, cerebrospinal fluid smears from centrifuged material increases positivity. The examination of samples of the lower airways useful in the initial treatment of pneumonia. . A sample of respiratory submit, primarily polymorphonuclear inflammatory cells should be cultivated way,

Direct examination using specific and special stains, it is useful in the diagnosis of diseases caused by M. tuberculosis, Bordetella pertussis, Francisella tularensis, Legionella pneumophila jirovesi pneumonia, Chlamydia and Plasmodium.

SENSITIVITY infecting organism

His determination should only be performed on pure cultures of microorganisms, because the results of the mixed cultures can provide wrong information or also have the disadvantage that their results are not obtained until 36- 48h after the initial sample was taken.

One of the most common methods for bacterial antimicrobial susceptibility is the disk diffusion method, for its ease of implementation, low cost and providing data within a 18- 24h. However, it is only semi-quantitative and is not useful in the case of microorganisms growth slow and difficult; plus it has not been properly standardized with respect to anaerobic bacteria. Their results are reported in terms of: sensitive, intermediate and resistant, the latter indicating that under certain circumstances antimicrobials may inhibit the detection microorganism in question.

Quantitative data on sensitivity are determined by broth microdilution techniques or Aggar, which the lowest concentration of antimicrobial agent that prevents visible growth after incubation for 18-24h. [Minimum inhibitory concentration (MIC)]. It is generally considered that a microorganism is sensitive when the MIC is at least a quarter of the peak serum concentration that is easily obtained with the antimicrobial. These methods also speaks of other important concepts such as: Minimum Bactericidal Concentration (MBC) or minimum lethal concentration

It is important to recognize the fact that susceptibility testing and clinical judgment requiring interpretation. They also identify resistant subpopulations, which is very important when resistance to an antimicrobial is caused by an enzyme that is normally repressed in the absence of such a product.

The indications for monitoring serum antimicrobial differ depending on the product and clinical situations. In general, systematically monitor these levels is not justified. This applies especially to patients who are well tolerated antimicrobial and infection responds quickly, or conversely, monitoring may be useful in selected patients whose infection persists despite treatment, symptoms and signs suggestive of toxicity or cases where drugs are used with a narrow margin between therapeutic efficacy value and toxicity;as happens with aminoglycosides.

SEROLOGICAL TESTS

Serodiagnosis is based on the principle that what aminoglycosides.,the reaction between an antigen and an antibody that can cause an event to register.

Although over the years the techniques have been refined, the aims pursued remain without changes: Identifying Antigen (Ag) or an Antibody (Ab) to help determine the aetiological importance of the particular microorganism and measuring the immune response thereto. It should be clarified that the results of these tests alone seldom sufficient to establish the diagnosis. In addition, a single determination of antibodies has little value because it does not provide indication of the timing of infection and had to be increased to four times the title between acute and convalescent sample to confirm the presence of infection

Interpretation of a particular method serodiagnóstico should be based on two important concepts:

- **Sensitivity:** A measure of the ability of a method to be positive in people known to have the disease..

- Specifically: It is a reflection of the ability of the test to be negative in individuals they do not suffer the disease.

With the improvement of neutralization tests, together with the development of fluorescent antibody techniques and hoping to achieve effective Viral chemotherapy, Serodiagnosis of viral diseases is called to achieve in the near future, a increasingly important role.

However, in the bacterial field, few advances made; except venereal diseases and bacterial meningitis, probably because bacteria can quickly and safely identified with cultivation techniques.

Inmunoabsorventes Advances in enzyme-linked tests to detect bacterial antigens by enzyme-labeled antibodies are promising and already commercially available for several reagents. However, bacterial field, few advances made; except for venereal disease and bacterial meningitis, probably because the bacteria can quickly and safely identify with cultivation techniques.

Reference

• Pediatric Infectious Diseases. Lactam resistance to bacteria.

Gram positive Vol. IV Norteam Clin Med, 1997.

• Basic Laboratory Procedures in Clinical bacteriology. 2d ed. Ed. McGraw-Hill, 7548-7855, 2003.

• KF Widmann clinical interpretation of laboratory tests. Ed. Revolutionary, 1989.

• Llop H. Valdes-Dapena V. Ma. M. Medical Microbiology and Parasitology Ed. Ecimed. Volume I. 81-99, 2001.

• Murray PR Medical microbiology. The 4th ed. Ed. Mosby. Vol. 4: 195-395, 2002.

• Frobischer M. Microbiology. Madrid: Salvat Editores SA, 1969.

• Appelbaum PC, Cli Bozdogan B. Lab Med. 24,381,2004.

• V. Lorian Antibiotics in Laboratory Medicine. Five edition, Ed Williams & Wilkins, Baltimore, 2000.

• Behrman RE, Kliegman RM, Jenson B H. Nelson. Treaty of Pediatrics, 17th edition. Ed. Elseiver, 2004

• Gilbert ND, Moellering RC, Sande A M. The Sanford. Guide to Antimicrobial Therapy. Thirty-one Edition, 2004.

• Organization. World   Health Manual   of   Biosafety   in the laboratory. Third edition. WHO, Geneva, 2005.

• Transport of Infectious subtances. Geneva, Word Health organization, 2004 (http://www.who.int/csr/resources/publications/WHO-CDS-CSR-LYO-2004-9/en/).

• Furr A K. CPR handbook of laboratory safety, 5th ed. Boca Raton, FL, CRC Press, 2000.

• Courvalin P, Goldstein F, Philippon A, Sirot J. L'antibiogramme. Editions MPC-Videom, parís, Bruxelles, 1987.

- Schunemann HJ, Oxman AD, Brozek J, et al. Grading quality of evidence and strength of recommendations for diagnostic tests and strategies. *Bmj.* May 17 2008;336(7653):1106-1110.

- Del Castillo Martín F, Lodoso Torrecilla B, Baquero Artigao F, García Miguel MJ, de José Gómez MI, Aracil Santos FJ, et al. Incremento de la incidencia de neumonía bacteriana entre 2001 y 2004. An Pediatr (Barc) 2008; 68: 99-102.

- Calbo E, Díaz A, Canadell E, Fabrega J, Uriz S, Xercavins M, et al. Invasive pneumococcal disease among children in a health district of Barcelona: early impact of pneumococcal conjugate vaccine. Clin Microbiol Infect 2006; 12 (9): 867-72.

- Obando I, Arroyo LA, Sánchez-Tatay D, Tarrago D, Moreno D, Hausdorff WP, et al. Molecular epidemiology of paediatric invasive pneumococcal disease in southern Spain after the introduction of heptavalent pneumococcal conjugate vaccine. Clin Microbiol Infect 2007; 13 (3): 347-8.

Chapter   6

ANTIMICROBIAL USE POLICY

The use of antimicrobials should be scientific and rational, that is, responsible. Medical staff plays an important role with their knowledge and experience. However, its application is not without problems.

Studies on the subject have detected differences in consumption by countries, regions and institutions, as well as deficiencies related to their prescription

- Excessive use
- inadequate selection,
- dose time and route of incorrect administration
- Appearance of preventable adverse effects
- inappropriate combinations
- Lack of resistance patterns
- Little or no use of procedures to monitor their effectiveness.

The prescription and consumption trends can be influenced by many factors including physician preferences, availability of medicine and even propaganda of the pharmaceutical industry.

Many countries have implemented national drug policies in order to ensure quality of care. Cuba is no exception. . In 1996 the Ministry of Public Health applies the strategy of pharmacoepidemiology, one of the five basic strategies that are designed and implemented for years in the national health system

The main purposes of this strategy are:

- To describe patterns of prescribing medications establish policies for selecting and using the same.

- Identify suboptimal therapeutic practices to develop actions of medical and regulatory education.

- Create a permanent structure therapy training and provide updated information on drugs to prescribers information.

- Promote and coordinate research drug utilization and pharmacoepidemiology to know the reality and measure the impact of interventions.

As can be seen, the antimicrobial policies are part of this national strategy designed and implemented.

Conceptually, the term policy in one of its meanings means "the art of Driving a matter to an end ", from the point of view of antimicrobials it is defined as the set of activities or tasks performed by a multidisciplinary group of professionals, with the objective of achieving rational use of these medicines in an institution and therefore, help reduce bacterial resistance.

The most difficult task to implement a policy of antimicrobial medical staff is aware of its necessity ... The prescription of antimicrobials carried out by doctors it is the result of a number of considerations and decisions regarding the course of a disease and the role that plays in drug treatment. In each prescription they reflected: the drugs available, information has been spread about them (which has come to the doctor and he has played) and the conditions under which conducts medical process.

Prescribing is a deductive logic, based on a comprehensive and objective information about the health problem presented by the patient. It should not be considered as a reflex, a recipe or a response to commercial pressures. After established the definitive diagnosis requires a clinical exercise intelligence to assess what is the best treatment strategy (pharmacological or not), of all the possible alternatives.

The rational use of antimicrobials involves getting the best effect with the least possible number of drugs for a short period of time and at reasonable cost.

The right choice of an antimicrobial should be made taking into account the criteria of efficacy, safety, convenience, cost. It should provide an appropriate treatment regimen, according to the individual characteristics of the patient to facilitate compliance with the prescription.

If important is making the decision to start one, most important therapy is still determined to ensure appropriate follow our prescribing behavior and plan a systematic evaluation not only of the clinical course of the disease, but the consequences of such treatment (risk-benefit ratio) in actual clinical practice.

Once sensitized physicians to the need to implement the policy of antimicrobials, start it the most important task is to obtain maps or reports microbiological presence and strength of the institution. Other equally important activities are the creation of a technical advisory group, the categorization of antimicrobials: Controlled, Semi-controlled and restricted or booking. Develop internal or treatments for conditions (choice and alternatives) in each service guidelines, which may not coincide with those in the literature and are not static because they depend on the situation of bacterial resistance to every place and every moment specific. Finally, it is necessary to apply systematic educational and training plans and implement the monitoring of its implementation.

Antimicrobials are a resource that should go only when they are really needed. The present and future to face the immense versatility of the bacteria in their quest for survival strategy can not rest solely on the ingenuity of researchers to create superior antimicrobial, they should also be used correctly and the measures taken to avoid transmission multiresistant microorganisms.

ASPECTS TO EVALUATE TO IMPOSE antimicrobial treatment

In the first chapter of this review established that made it successful treatment in infectious diseases dependent on a complex process where many factors interact with each other. Let's look in more detail these and other factors related:

1. DEPENDENT FACTORS CAUSING AGENT

- **Microorganism type:**

In medicine, the term is reserved for pathogens that which is capable of producing disease. In the field of infections they are plentiful (bacteria, viruses, fungi, protozoa and helminths). Bacteria, besides being a heterogeneous group, cause more infections than other microorganisms-.It is therefore essential, before imposing a treatment,antimicrobial determine whether the bacteria is: Gram positive or Gram negative
- aerobic or anaerobic

- **Sensitivity :**

Knowledge of the in vitro susceptibility of the causative agent through susceptibility is necessary to impose an effective antimicrobial treatment. This allows to know the suitability of one or more antimicrobials for the treatment of a particular infection-.
Likewise this study provides important information about:

Minimal inhibitory concentration (MIC) of the antimicrobial concentration capable of inhibiting the proliferation or growth of the strain studied(MBC).

Minimum bactericidal concentration The concentration at which the death of the microorganism antimicrobials causes.

These elements are useful for dispensing Meet or exceed the MIC is sufficient to treat the majority of infections. Reach the CBM would only be justified in cases of serious infections.

- Resistance

This aspect has already been widely discussed (see Chapter 2). However it is important to make it clarified that it is not the same resistance that sensitivity.
When a pathogen can multiply in the presence of an antimicrobial that was previously sensitive is because it has been changed or has acquired new properties that allow it to resist its action .
A microorganism is regarded insensitive because it lacks the target site that allows the antimicrobial perform its action.
Resistant pathogens are not more virulent than sensitive, but are more difficult to remove.
In the hospital environment is where most frequently develops resistance and one of the major causes has been the use of broad-

spectrum antimicrobial when a narrow spectrum can be effective, or use unnecessarily long subtherapeutic doses or treatments.

- ### Kinetics **growth**

  The microorganisms that multiply slowly are less sensitive to antimicrobial action of the rapid multiplication.

  The classic example is Mycobacterium tuberculosis that multiplies rapidly in caves intermittently in cheesyfoci and slowly within macrophages. Therefore, the effectiveness of the treatment will depend on using a combination of antimicrobial drugs able to have activity against the three cell populations, which could not be achieved with monotherapy.

2. Antimicrobial FACTORS

Most factors evaluated in this regard have already been described earlier in this book (see Chapter 1). However, others want to address here are no less important and deserve special attention:

- ### **Empirical antimicrobial Whether or not**

  the first decision the doctor must make is to determine whether administration of the antimicrobial is indicated or not.

  If it is then we must make the right selection.
  Of course, most of the time we do not have all the elements we have described to identify the causative agent and we are in the dilemma of imposing an antimicrobial treatment empirically, which in no way It means it is unscientific.

  The empirical treatment is warranted when when imposing treatment agent either ignored because it is not possible to study or do not have the results and initiation of treatment can not be delayed.

  Outside these reasons it is better to wait and start specific treatment once the causative organism identified Post-antibiotic.

- ### **Effect**

  On several occasions, antimicrobials are administered according to an intermittent regimen, so many periods occur during which no antimicrobial present in tissues or body fluids and yet established chemotherapy remains effective.

Eagle demonstrated this phenomenon many years ago when he reported that many Gram positive organisms again not proliferate for several hours after exposure to penicillin, a fact that now it is known as Post Antibiotic Effect. That is, although not all infective microorganisms are eradicated, they do not proliferate again for several hours after exposure to a concentration above the MIC.

Virtually all antimicrobials exhibit this effect against Gram positive microorganisms, but only somewhat They presented against Gram negative bacteria. Aminoglycosides and the new quinolones (norfloxacin, ofloxacin and ciprofloxacin) show this effect against Gram positive and negative bacteria.

It has also been seen that in the phase of post-antibiotic exposure microorganisms are more sensitive to killing by leukocytes.

- **Combinations of antimicrobial drugs:**

Ideally, use a single antimicrobial whenever possible. Some exceptions in very severe cases, combinations of antimicrobials are no more effective than treatment with a single drug.

In cases where the combination of antimicrobials is required to keep in mind that the situation and the medical decision could seriously complicate It .why it is important to know the possible effects of combinations of antimicrobials, as it is a prerequisite when the indication of proper medical treatment

Classically four major effects of these associations are known antimicrobial

a) Synergy: This effect is when two antimicrobials that act in different sites of the bacterial cell and the result is the multiplication of their actions are combined. Example penicillins and aminoglycosides addition.

b) Summation and / or It is the sum of the action of an antimicrobial compound with another. It occurs when antimicrobials having the same action mechanism is used. Example: Penicillin and Cephalosporins.

c) Competition   It manifests when two are used, two antimicrobials whose mechanisms of action are different (bacteriostatic bactericidal), but the action does not help one another, winning the competition on the bactericidal bacteriostatic. Example: penicillins and tetracyclines. Remember that the bactericidal effect of an antimicrobial is manifested to a greater extent against rapidly growing germs. Yes bacteriostatic associates whose mechanism of action is to reduce pathogen multiplication, establish a competition that affect the bactericidal effect of the former

.
d) Antagonism When two antimicrobial agents which provide a much smaller effect combine that would produce (the agent, of them, more effective) if used alone. . Example: Cycloserine with Tetracycline or

Chloramphenicol combinations or frequent use of broad-spectrum antimicrobial covers the diagnostic inaccuracy, provides a false sense of security and has the following disadvantages:

- Increased cost of treatment
- Increased rate of superinfection
- Increased of antimicrobial resistant bacteria
- Increased adverse reactions due to interactions
- Appearance of antagonisms between antimicrobial success.

• **Pharmacokinetics:**

Know the processes of absorption, distribution, biotransformation and excretion of antimicrobials is very valuable in the treatment .
The route of administration is dependent on the absorption and the severity of the infection. In severe infections parenteral route is used: EV slow or continuous infusion. In mild to moderate infections can start with the mouth and if the absorption of the drug in this way is optimal.
Not forget that in some cases administration with food reduced the oral bioavailability as with tetracyclines. The Tissue distribution of antimicrobial depends on many factors such as lipid solubility, plasma protein binding, tissue or organ perfusion where the infection is located, etc.
The antimicrobial with little binding to plasma proteins are
widely distributed, although there are exceptions such as aminoglycosides , although little is bound to plasma proteins, their molecular size makes its distribution in the body is reduced.
The biotransformation can occur in the liver (phenicols, macrolides, nitroimidazoles Lincosamides), others do kidney, intestine ; some become active metabolites, while others are inactivated in this process.

Its excretion may be through the kidney only (chloramphenicol, sulfonamides, nitrofurantoin and vancomycin) or kidney and bile duct (beta-lactams, aminoglycosides, quinolones, . tetracyclines, lincosamides and Rifamycines), although the latter, in case of obstruction, reduces the effectiveness of antimicrobial

- **Dosage and duration of treatment:**

The most frequent errors in antimicrobial therapy are dose-related, the intervals between them, as well changes to be made no later than 48 hours after starting the administration, without justification for doing so.

The dose can not be determined at fixed terms, therefore dose ranges are used. It is equally damaging the defect excess dosing. Let's see what happens in two cases:
- If we double the dose or increase the frequency of administration we can approach toxic levels that can be dangerous, especially if the antimicrobial has a narrow margin of safety doubled.
- If administering half the dose or intervals, the serum level of the drug away from the CIM which may cause failures in the treatment and promote bacterial resistance.

As for the duration of treatment, usually suffice for 3 to 5 days to observe the onset of the beneficial effect of antimicrobial. If no adequate response to the expiration of the minimum time should be considered a change of antimicrobial, they must first be ruled out possible causes that hinder its action.
An excessively prolonged treatment increases the possibility of adverse effects, emergence of resistance and costs.

3. DEPENDENT FACTORS host

- **Infection Location:**

Generally, in the well-perfused tissues accessible and higher tissue concentrations are obtained and in which are inaccessible as eye, bones, meninges local instillation may be required in addition to systemic administration.
The deterioration of the circulation or ischemia can affect the arrival of antimicrobials to the focus of infection

Meningeal inflammation may increase concentrations of the drug at this level

- **Policies focus**

  The presence of pus, the acidic environment may promote or hypoxic inactivation of antimicrobials (aminoglycosides, glycopeptides), others like tetracyclines and nitrofurantoin are more active in acid medium.
  A foreign body (joint prostheses, heart valves, catheter, indwelling urethral biliary or kidney stones) may interfere with the antimicrobial action, because the microorganisms accumulate on the surface and covered with a layer of glycocalyx that protects leukocytes and the antimicrobial agent.

COMMON CAUSES OF Antimicrobial FAILURE

THE ORGANISM:

  a) Development of resistance
  b) initially dual infection (detecting and treating only one)
  c) superinfection
  d) Reporting wrong susceptibility of the organism

2. Antimicrobial:

  inadequate a) Selection
  b) Route of administration and inadequate doses
  c) level in blood and inadequate tissue (malabsorption, Local inactivation, etc.)

3. PATIENT:
  a) undrained abscess pus
  b) infected or retained foreign body
  c) Immunodeficiency

With all these elements is possible to establish an adequate institutional antimicrobial policy that would ensure proper use of these drugsPeña.

Reference

Cabrera LN, M. M, Cires M. P, Acosta GJ behavior of resistance in vitro following a policy of antimicrobials. Rev Cubana Hig Epidem. 1993; 31 (2):. 100-108

García SJ Criteria for the implementation of a policy of antibiotics in hospitals. Cuban Rev Public Health 1991; 17 (2): 74-78 microbiology..

Murray PR Medical The 4th ed. Ed. Mosby. Vol. 4: 195-395, 2002.

Goodman and Bilman. Pharmacological Basis of Therapeutics. Vol II ed 9 (2):1996.

Monthly. Over antibiotic us. Prescribing references. Ed. Sales-Sataff. 188-208, 2005.

Jawetz E et al. Medical microbiology. 15th ed. Mexico City Ed. TheManual ModernSA, 1996.

Rudolph H. Antibacterial therapy.20th ed. Ed. Appleton and Lange. 444, 1996.

Llop H. Valdes-Dapena V. Ma. M. Medical Microbiology and Parasitology Ed. Ecimed. Volume I. 81-99, 2001.

MSD Group. Antibacterial drugs. Merck Sharp & Dohme of Spain. SA 2000 [INTERNET (http: jeffline.tju.edu/cuis/oac/antibiotics- guide / /into.htlm)]

MINSAP Centre for the Development of pharmacoepidemiology Formulary.. National Cuba, 2003.

Chapter 7

PROPER HANDLING OF ANTIMICROBIAL

Choosing the right antimicrobial for treatment of an infection is a daily problem for the doctor either community-acquired or nosocomial faces., The clinician should know and appreciate the interaction between the three factors involved in the infection process: microorganism, patient and drug. (Figure 1)

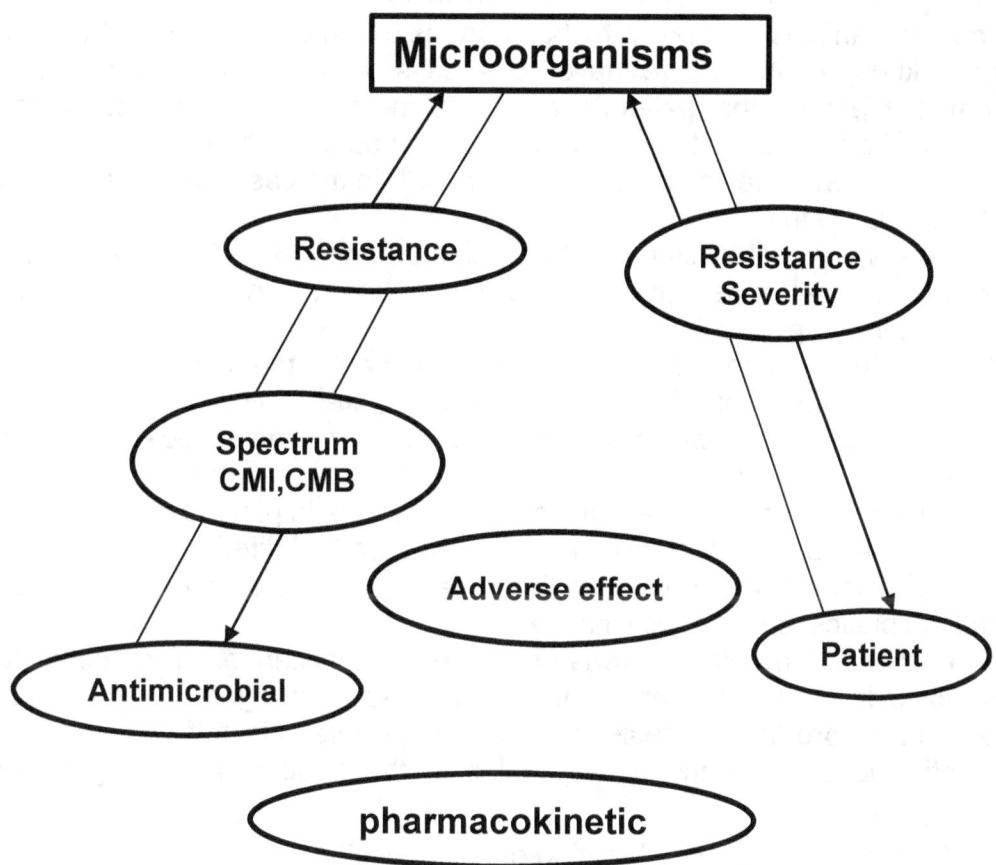

MIC: Minimum Inhibitory Concentration
MBC: Minimum Bactericidal Concentration

Figure 1: Relationship between the three intervening factors involved in infection.

The choice of antibiotic treatment is not easy, in relation to the proliferation of antibiotics emerged in the last the changing patterns of resistance of different microorganisms and increasingly complex diagnosis of infectious processes. Which makes difficult the choice of empirical antibiotic treatment especially if the patient has received prior antibiotic treatment. This problem requires compliance with antibiotic policies outside and inside the hospital treatment.

The clinician should ask the following questions before choosing an empirical antibiotic

Does the patient really an infection? An antibiotic treatment based on clinical findings indicated? Is it an emergency situation?

And even being an infection, the most common cause of infections in pediatric patients are viral.

Are obtained, examined and appropriate clinical specimens grown?

What microorganisms are likely to be responsible infection? Does the local microflora known? Should we have to assess whether the community or nosocomial infection, the patient's age, the most common microorganism according to the location of the focus, Boasts the use of antibiotics, the immune status of the patient. The valuation of a Gram CSF in the case of infection of the central nervous system.

If you have several antibiotics to treat the microorganism Which one is right? Is the pattern of local sensitivity and resistance known? Are there empirical antibiotic treatment protocols?

The choice of the right antibiotic is going to be related to the suspected etiology and major infectious problems community-acquired or nosocomial. The existence of empirical antibiotic treatment protocols promote decision making and therapeutic uniformity.

Rate kinetics and dynamics of antibiotic concentrations in plasma and source of infection, post-antibiotic effect, protein binding, serum half-life.

Economic considerations. Professionals increasingly we are forced to use more powerful antibiotics, broad spectrum and

costs in connection with increased bacterial resistance. The costs of antimicrobial drugs are an important part of hospital budgets. This problem coupled with the proliferation resistance of germs is essential fulfilling

policy antibiotic and therapeutic strategies in the hospital according to the situation the same.

- Is it reasonable for a combination of antibiotics?

On matching diseases life threatening patients using bactericidal antibiotics and spread spectrum principle recommended. The synergy has proved useful in septic patients of unknown etiology and in neutropenic. Avoid not synergistic partnerships that can foster the antagonism between them and the treatment failure and the emergence of resistant strains therapy.

Situations that can be used combined

1. Empirical treatment of polymicrobial infections should be chosen different antimicrobials with different spectra to expand activity against all microorganisms that may be involved, as in the abdominal, liver, brain, etc.abscesses.
2. Treatment of severe sepsis by unknown agents.
3. To achieve synergistic effect and / or decrease the emergence of resistance.
4. To increase the therapeutic effect of each antimicrobial, by itself, to promote more rapid and complete bactericidal effect that helps reduce the days of treatment or dose reduction of one or both antimicrobials but the therapeutic effect is similar.
5. To prevent enzyme inactivation of antimicrobial, making sensitive to producing microorganisms destroying enzymes (beta-lactamases.)
6. To reduce the side effects of more effective agent.

- Are host factors must be taken into account specific considerations regarding?

- The immune status of the host, as well as kidney and liver function, are important factors to consider, circumstances They should be taken into account when choosing antibiotics with hepatorenal toxicity. In situations where host defenses are compromised, immunosuppressed, leucopenic patients with fever, etc., is well established administration of several antibiotics in the empirical antimicrobial therapy.

- What is the best route of administration? What is the proper dosage?

  The proper dosage will be established, keeping the interval between them according to the pharmacokinetic properties of antibiotic. It is useful to determine serum concentrations, in order to achieve the best therapeutic effect and reduce toxic effects.

- A modification will be necessary in the initial treatment after bacteriological results?

  After 72 hours of initiation of treatment, We should make a review of empirical antimicrobial treatment in relation to the clinical course and bacteriological results, treatment should be geared according to these.

- What is the optimal duration of treatment? Is it likely to show resistance and / or toxic effects?

  The optimal duration of antibiotic treatment will be in accordance with the type of infectious disease, patient advocacy mechanisms, underlying disease and its possible toxic effects. Prolongation associated with a risk of superinfection by fungi and increased resistance.

Reasons why the indiscriminate use of antimicrobials.

- diagnostic errors.
- inadequate antibiotic prophylaxis indication
- Complacency
- Consider resistance and virulence as similar concepts

Consequences antimicrobial resistance

- Increased mortality from infectious diseases
- Increased morbidity criticism.
- Increased hospital costs
- threatens to undermine the effectiveness of the programs of health care.

After the discovery and the widespread use sulfa drugs and penicillin in the mid-twentieth century, the period between 1950 and 1970 was the "golden age" of discovery of antibiotics. It was possible to treat and cure many serious and sometimes life-threatening infections. However, these successes encouraged the overuse and misuse of antibiotics. Currently, many microorganisms have acquired resistance to different antibiotics and, in some cases, nearly all. Knowledge of the most common germs in each type of IRAM and sensitivity patterns help us to schedule a rational use of empirical antibiotics.

Resistant bacteria can cause increased morbidity and death, particularly in patients with serious underlying disease or immunodeficiency. Antimicrobial resistance is a problem for hospitals, transmission of bacteria is enhanced because of the high vulnerability of the population. And propagation resistance among bacteria is usually the result of selection pressure by antibiotics. Resistant bacteria are transmitted from one patient to another and resistance factors are transferred from one bacterium to another and both occur more frequently in health care facilities. Continued use of antimicrobials increases selection pressure favoring the emergence, growth and spread of resistant strains. They are contributing factors to this uncontrolled and inappropriate use of antimicrobial agents, including excessive prescription of suboptimal doses administration, the short duration of treatment and misdiagnosis leading to inappropriate medication selection. In health care facilities, the spread of resistant organisms is facilitated when there best practices hand washing, care is exercised by placing barriers and cleaning of equipment. The emergence of resistance also contributes administering insufficient doses by shortages of antibiotics, where the lack of microbiology laboratories leads to the empirical prescription and where the lack of other agents increases the risk of treatment failure.

The importance of microbial map for each specific unit is what gives guidance on the use of one or another antibiotic depending on the sensitivity shown by microbiology either its minimum inhibitory concentration or methods of qualitative confrontation.

In reviewing the international literature, the 50s is known as "the era of Staphylococcus" because so far they were susceptible to penicillin evenly, gradually began to develop resistance mediated by beta-lactamases, especially the phage 80-81. This germ can be regarded as a paradigm of "hospital pathogen." Their emergence coincided with the increasingly widespread use of broad-spectrum antibiotics. In the early 60s, staphylococci pandemic began to decline related to the introduction of new antibiotics resistant to beta-lactamases that were effective against Staphylococcus. These multidrug resistant germs are an example of the old adage that "yesterday saprophytes pathogens are today," it is now known to cause catheter-related, vascular prostheses, surgical wound infection and bacteremia. Although none of the species resistant staphylococci seems to be more virulent than those sensitive, the fact multidrug resistance involves a major drug spending.

Studies demonstrate the increase in this agent as an important seed in sepsis and with great impact on the resistance of nosocomial strains. Whenever an antimicrobial is introduced, resistance develops. The hospital is the ideal habitat for pathogens whatever their variety, each day expose more powerful resistance to antimicrobials. The "intensive" use of antibiotic s seriously distorts the endogenous microflora of the patient and eventually favored colonization and infection with multi-resistant germs.

The highest frequency of antimicrobial resistant which is of deep concern to the medical community microorganisms. It occurs when health workers become transient carriers to take them in his hands.

OMS measures to contain antimicrobial resistance

In the population and prescribers of AMB

• Education programs for the population.

• Ensure that prescribers have access to authoritative documentation on your prescription.

In Hospitals

• Create Committees therapeutic drug that can monitor the use of antibiotics

• Develop and regularly update treatment protocols
AMB

• Ensuring the availability of microbiological laboratory by type of hospital

• Promote and control measures for control and prevention of infection in the Hospital

• Handwashing

• Comply with hospital isolation measures

REFERENCES

1. Caballero López. Intensive therapy; the 1st ed. Editorial Medical Sciences, 2009; 1631-1633.
2. Richard E. Beherman, MD. Antibiotics. In Handbook of Pediatrics Nelson; The 1st ed. American Ed., 2002; 813 to 817.884.
3. F. Ruza. Rational Use of Antibiotics. Pharmacological Basis and Farmadinámicas. Rn Treaty Pediatric Intensive Care, 3rd ed. Standard editions - Capital. 2003; 1586-1594.
4. Nosocomial infections INTERHOSPITAL rates for comparison: limitations and possible solutions - A report from NNIS System. Infect Control Hosp Epidemiol. 2008; 10: 123-45.
5. Caballero, JM Cisneros, R. Luque Cansed Comparative Study of bacteremia by Enterococcus spp. With and without high-level Resistance to Vancomicyn. J Clin Microbiol. 2007; 19 (2): 39-42.
6. LL Dever. China C, Eng HK, Debnovan C, Johanson WG. Vancomicyn-resitant Enterococcus in childrens in a Medical Center. Association with antibiotic usage.AJIC. 2008; 26 (4): 40-6.
7. Brooks G, Butel J, Nicholas O. Medical Microbiology Jawet z JY J. Melnick E. Adelberg Med Havana. ECIMED; 2006.
8. Rodney D, W. Costenton Biofilms: Survival Mechanisms of Clinically Relevant microorganism. Clin Microbiol Rev.2007; 1: 16-34.
9. Walsh That Antibiotics act on cell wall biosynthesis, In: Antibiotics actions, origins, resistance. Washington DC. Am Soc Microbiol. 2006; 20-41.
10. Estrada B. meticillin -resistant staphylococcus in the Community. Infect Med. 2007; 18 (13): 435-46.
11. Rogues AM, Dumartin C, Amadeo B, Venier AG, Marty N, P Parneix, Gachie JP. Relationship Between rates of antimicrobial consumption and the incidence of antimicrobial resistance in Staphylococcus aureus and Pseudomonas aeruginosa isolates from 47 French hospitals. Infect Control Hosp Epidemiol. 2007 Dec; 28 (12): 1389-1395.
12. Paterson DL. The role of antimicrobial management programs in optimizing antibiotic prescribing Within hospitals. Clin Infect Dis 2006 Jan 15; 42 Suppl 2: S90-S95.
13. Fica CA, MA Hair, Juliet LC, DP Prado, Bavestrello F L. Among Intravenous antimicrobial use different hospital in Chile During 2005 Rev Chilena Infectol. 2008 Dec; 25 (6): 419-27.
14. Beovic B, Kreft S, K Seme, Cizman M. The impact of total control of antibiotic prescribing by infectious disease specialist on antibiotic consumption and cost. J Chemother. 2009 Feb; 21 (1): 46-51.

Chapter 8

ANTIMICROBIAL IN UNITS Pediatric Intensive Care

One of the most common choices for the intensivist wielding admitted critically ill patients is choosing the right antimicrobial to treat an infection, either community-acquired or nosocomial.

It is known that depending on the type of Pediatric Intensive Care Unit (PICU) is polyvalent or surgical, severity of patients, pathology, etc., more than 80% of patients receiving one or more antimicrobial and some authors argue that about 50% of these treatments antimicrobials taxes are recognized in subsequent valuations, they were not justified in relation to the existence of a bacterial infection process base, but were due to other causes of systemic inflammatory response syndrome (SIRS) noninfectious, Central, tumor, drug fever, low output situation, etc.

If at any time it becomes difficult this decision is in the east, where most of the time the intensivist has to face not only the points raised in the preceding chapters, but derivatives also increasingly complex diagnosis of infectious processes, especially in patients admitted to hospital with suspected nosocomial infection and severe pathology, in chronic cases, subjected to invasive diagnostic and therapeutic procedures and the Most of the time, and has received several antimicrobial previously.

Added to this it is that, even most of the time, the antimicrobial treatment of choice must be empirical, as the severity of symptoms this does not augur more specific confirmatory results. Then comes the dilemma born of doubt and the hard choice.

Dealing with this situation it requires adherence to a policy of antibiotics in the hospital, with the acceptance of previously agreed measures, where the service design collective strategies according to the particular situation of each hospital.

Elements themselves NOSOCOMIAL INFECTION IN CHILDREN

1. Severity is related not only with the pathogen, but also with age in relation to its worst immune response.
2. The predominant nosocomial pathogens are aerobic Gram positive.
3. The most common infection is nosocomial catheter-related bacteremia, respiratory infection followed and, finally, urinary tract infection.
4. There is increased risk of bacteremia and high mortality rates with infectious secondary locations (meningitis).

ELEMENTS TO BE CONSIDERED FOR Empirical Antimicrobial Therapy

To establish an empirical antimicrobial therapy should be considered the following

- Circumstances:.Location of the infectious process

- Ecology Bacterial.

- Patterns of resistance in the intensive care unit.

- Severity of the underlying disease.

Patient's immune status.

- Previous use of antimicrobials.

- Adequacy functioning of organs and systems.

- Possible interactions with other drugs.

- Hospital stay

- Special Situations (existence of prosthesis, catheterizations, aggressive procedures, etc.)

Definitions:

Phlebitis:
Presence of inflammatory signs of multiple causes in or around the site of insertion of intravascular device infection.

b) Catheter-related :
Presence of microorganisms in any segment of the catheter
(determined by quantitative or semi-quantitative methods) bacteremia.

c) Catheter-related

Presence of the same microorganisms in a segment of the catheter and the blood culture sepsis.

d) Catheter-related

Presence same germ in the catheter and blood cultures also associated with signs of systemic inflammatory response.

ASSESSMENT OF RISK FACTORS

- Extreme ages of life (newborn)

- Alterations of defense mechanisms (immune)

- Severity underlying disease

- Outbreaks of infection varied

- Staphylococcal colonization

- Longer hospital stays of 14 days (modification of the flora)

- Parenteral nutrition

- Type catheter

- Place insertion site:
  - Femoral (area easy contamination)
  - Antecubital (preferred area)
  - Jugular or subclavian

- Insertion technique

- Catheterization duration (no more than 7-8 days usually)

- Integration of urgency (justified violation of the rules of aseptic and antiseptic)

- Dilution and rate of infusion of drugs.

- Care catheter.

FREQUENTLY etiological agents:

- In local infections:
  Germs Gram positive affect 51%
  - Germs Gram negative affect 41%

- mixed seeds affecting 30%
- Fungi affect 2%

- In systemic infections:
  - Gram positive germs affect 63%
  - Germs Gram negative affect 28%
  - mixed seeds affecting 12%
  - Fungi affect 6%

SURVEILLANCE catheter infection:

a) Conducting Skin cultures:
- Before insertion
- During insertion
- After insertion

b) Making catheter cultures and blood of the patient:
- the cap
- the outer coupling
- blood Blood culture
- Gram of the catheter tip

c) inspection of the insertion site for signs of infection

Complications

LOCAL 1):
- Pleural effusion and empyema
- Pneumatoceles
- Pneumothorax
- Atelectasis
- Pulmonary edema
- Pronchopleural fistulas
- Pulmonary abscess

2) Systemic:
- Extrapulmonary infection focus from Pneumonic (myocarditis, meningoencephalitis, etc.)
- Sepsis and / or Severe sepsis

- Septic shock

FACTORS TO EVALUATE THE START OF PNEUMONIA hospital Antimicrobial Therapy:

- Place where it was acquired:
  - Open hospitalization or UTIP
- previous Conditions of Patient:
  - Non infectious or infectious (respiratory or breathing)
- Underlying disease:
  - Congenital heart disease
  - Asthma
  - Neurological diseases
  - haematological disorders
  - Immunosuppression
- Use of antimicrobials prior used.
- hospital stay
- invasive procedures
  - Mechanical ventilation
  - nasogastric intubation
  - venous Approaches
  - Surgical interventions
- microbial Map techniques..
- Microbiological studies patient

Meningitis with no evidence of detectable bacterial pathogen in CSF by standard laboratory It was initially described as an acute syndrome with signs consistent with meningitis, pleocitosis, absence of bacteria in cultures of CSF and a relatively short and benign course. It is usually caused by viral infection, probably caused by enterovirus, adenovirus or herpes virus. Today, it covers a broad spectrum of infectious etiologies (viruses, mycobacteria, fungi) and noninfectious (malignancies, collagen, trauma, direct toxins, poisoning, drugs, autoimmune diseases, and others).

Partially treated Meningitis
It is the term which it may have caused more confusion when defining bacterial meningitis. Usually used to describe an infection of the central nervous system, patients receiving oral antibiotics prior to the time of diagnosis.

In this case, many authors think that antibiotics may cause changes in the values of cytochemical study cerebrospinal fluid of patients with signs or symptoms of meningitis, and that these changes may hinder the proper interpretation of the same, as the clinician may assume that the absence of the classical alterations of bacterial meningitis in the cytochemical, is due to prior receipt of antibacterial and not the fact that meningitis can be due to other causes. To this end we must clarify that upon receipt of antibiotics can only alter the Gram. or the result of the culture, but never cause cytochemical modifications.

Another important aspect to consider is that very few antibiotics administered orally achieved adequately penetrate the central nervous system and therefore sterilize the CSF. In this regard we should determine exactly what the patient has received antibiotic to know if it was or was not able to sterilize the cerebrospinal fluid, only in order to understand that the disease has not been identified in Gram or isolated in culture and not to explain cytochemical findings that are not compatible with bacterial meningitis. Finally, if the term were to be adequate in essence, patients should only complete specific therapy days missing from the time the diagnosis is made and not receive the full course of antibiotics as always.

In short this term should only used to refer to cases in which suspected bacterial meningitis, but have sterile cultures, possibly as a result of previously received antibiotic therapy; but in no case should guide the therapeutic approach to be used.

Lymphocytic bacterial Meningitis
The vast majority of patients with bacterial meningitis have typical findings in the cytochemical cerebrospinal fluid that identify with reasonable certainty the etiology of the process. Among the findings is the significant increase in the level of CSF cells, usually at the expense of polymorphonuclear. However, there are some cases in which the lifting cell count (sometimes not as intense) occurs but at the expense of lymphocytes or monocytes; and yet we are in the presence of bacterial meningitis and viral meningitis not, as would be logical to assume. In these cases, it helps to diagnose the elevated protein and decreased glucose in CSF. It can be seen in Salmonella, Listeria monocytogenes, Haemophilus influenzae type b and Streptococcus pneumoniae, among others

Etiology.

80% of the MEB are caused by the following pathogens:

- Haemophilus influenzae type b
- Neisseria meningitidis
- Streptococcus pneumoniae

TREATMENT:

Treatment the MEB starts immediately after diagnostic lumbar puncture (LP) or in cases with strong suspicion and are severely affected (which is contraindicated PL).

They must be chosen antimicrobials proven effectiveness against the most common etiologic agents ., in proper and correct management schemes in order to achieve a bactericidal activity that would eradicate the bacteria CSF dose

In selecting the most appropriate antimicrobial should necessarily be taken into consideration various aspects:

a) Knowledge of the characteristics pharmacokinetic and pharmacodynamic of antibiotics to be used.
b) Patient age.
c) The epidemiology of the zone in which is located. d) The local bacterial resistance patterns.
e) The utility may have some ancillary tests to guide therapy to be used

REFERENCES

1. Seidel S James, Jane Knapp F. Editors. American Academy of Pediatrics. Childhood Emergencies in the Office, Hospital and Community. Organizing Systems of care. 2nd edition. USA, 2000.

2. C Mark Rogers, Helfaer A Mark. Handbook of Pediatric Intensive

3. Care. 3rd edition. Ed. Lippincott Williams & Wilkins. USA, 1999.

4. A. Roa Jaime Bernal editor. Pediatric Emergency and Emergency

5. Ministry of Municipal Public Health, Municipality of Santiago de Cali

6. Colombia, 1996.

7. M Barkin Roger, P. Rosen Pediatric Emergency. Guide for outpatient treatment. 5th edition. Ed. Harcourt-Mosby.Madrid, Spain, 2000.

8. Jacqz-Aigrain Evelyn, Choonara Imti.Paediatric Clinical Pharmacology. Ed. Taylor & Francis. New York, USA, 2006.

9. Collective authors. Clinical Practice Guidelines Intensive

10. Pediatric Care.Volume I and II. Policy Editor. Havana 2001.

11. Riverón Quintana A, Martinez M, Rosas B. Guidelines Management of bacterial meningitis in children. Venezuelan files Childcare and pediatrics. 2003; 66 (3): 10-52 pneumoniae..

12. D Meli, Christen S, Leib S, M. Tauber Current concepts in the pathogenesis of meningitis Caused by Streptococcus Curr Opin Infect Dis 2002; 15:. 253-257

13. M Chowdhury, Tunkel A. Antibacterial Agents in infections of the

14. Central Nervous System. Infect Dis Clin North Am 2000; 14 (2): 391-

15. 408.

16. MJ López Ruiz Casado Flores J. Pediatric Emergency vital.Rev

17. Spanish pediatrics 1993; 39: 227-288 emergencies..

18. Married Flores J, Marin C. Barba pediatric Realities and challenges. Rev Spanish Pediatrics 2000; 53 (1): 39-61 Iannone.

19. K George Siberry, Robert The Harriet Lane Handbook. 15th edition. Ed. Mosby. 2000.

20. Task Force of the American College Care Medicine Society of Critical Care Medicine. Crit Care Med 1999; . 27: 39-66

21. American Academy of Pediatrics. Pediatric Clinical Practice Guidelines & Policies. A compendium of Evidence-based research of Pediatric Practice,5th edition, 2005.